The Diffusion of Influenza

The Diffusion of Influenza

Patterns and Paradigms

Gerald F. Pyle

Rowman & Littlefield
PUBLISHERS

ROWMAN & LITTLEFIELD

Published in the United States of America in 1986
by Rowman & Littlefield, Publishers
(a division of Littlefield, Adams & Company)
81 Adams Drive, Totowa, New Jersey 07512

Library of Congress Cataloging-in-Publication Data

Pyle, Gerald F.
  The diffusion of influenza.

  Includes index.

   1. Influenza—Statistics. 2. Influenza—History.
3. Medical geography. 4. Epidemiology. I. Title.
[DNLM: 1. Influenza—history. 2. Influenza—occurrence.
WC515 P996d]
RA644.I6P95   1986   614.5′18′09   86-1780
ISBN 0-8476-7429-0

88 87 86
10 9 8 7 6 5 4 3 2 1

Printed in the United States of America

Dedicated to the Memory
of
Russell Roy Pyle

Contents

Tables and Figures

Acknowledgments

The very nature of influenza and the different ways it spreads leads many to attempt to unravel some of the mysteries underlying the spatial diffusion of the disease. This has been happening since long before the invention of the printing press. Clearly, it has only been during this century that we have begun to understand mechanisms contributing to influenza diffusion. As with any scientific phenomenon, interest in this problem seems to rise and fall as a result of both major pandemics and significant medical discoveries. Thus, public interest in the spread of influenza crested in 1918 (The Great Pandemic), 1933 (the discovery of the virus), 1957 (Asian influenza), 1968 (Hong Kong influenza) and during the "Swine Flu Scare" of 1976. My own interests in the problem span two decades as a result of a general interest in the geography of disease diffusion; however, specific concerns about the "modern" influenza diffusion era can be traced to the National Inoculation Program of 1976. A preliminary investigation of major contributions to the influenza literature at that time convinced me that while some works containing aspects of diffusion of the disease had been accomplished by such outstanding scholars as Alexander Langmuir, Sir Charles Stuart-Harris, Alfred Crosby, W. I. B. Beavridge, and a few others, the best geographical exposition of the disease by the late 1970s was the analysis of Asian Flu (H2N2/ 1957) in England and Wales by John Hunter and Jonathan Young. I expanded an initial review of influenza studies somewhat in a chapter on general disease diffusion in *Applied Medical Geography* published in 1979, but I realized then that much more research and analysis needed to be performed in attempting to develop a truly comprehensive understanding of mechanisms contributing to periodic and sometimes explosive outbreaks of a disease still counted as one of the ten leading causes of death in the United States.

It is with a great deal of appreciation that I acknowledge the support of the National Science Foundation, Geography and Regional Science Division, for the support necessary to make this volume possible through two grants entitled "The Simulation of

Influenza Diffusion" during the periods 1979–81 and 1982–84. I am particularly appreciative of the encouragement and understanding of Barry Moriarty, then director of the Geography and Regional Science Program of the National Science Foundation.

The completion of this work can be viewed in retrospect as consisting of three phases. The first consisted of acquisition of the data necessary for comparative statistical analyses as well as an extensive review of the history of influenza. This phase was initiated at the University of Akron and continued at the University of North Carolina at Charlotte. During that period Dennis Bregman, now chief statistician at the Centers for Disease Control, was most cooperative and helpful in the acquisition of influenza data from the federal archives and more recent computer tapes. Brian Berry offered considerable assistance during that phase in the form of consultation on methods of data analysis and urban-based units of observation that did indeed prove to be the most meaningful in the final simulation procedures. I am indebted to Brian for that assistance, and for related design consultation over the past two decades. Larry Brown of the Ohio State University also served as a consultant during that period, and I appreciate the computer software that Larry supplied to the project.

The second phase of the project consisted of case studies of influenza data sets or narrative accounts from different epidemics, pandemics, and general time periods. Peter Haggett was of considerable assistance during the beginning of that phase as he consulted on analytical findings both in Charlotte, North Carolina, and north of London at Hemingford Grey. John Hunter also continued to add valuable assistance in evaluating some of the earlier analyses and some accomplished later during this phase. Irene Schulze of the St. Louis School University Medical Center, School of Medicine, proved to be valuable as a virological consultant during this time, and her contributions helped crystallize some of my understanding of properties of influenza viruses. Also during this phase, some intellectually enlightening collaboration with K. David Patterson, a noted medical historian, led to some interesting joint publications. Working with Patterson was a genuinely rewarding experience, and we are both particularly indebted to G. Melvyn Howe for cooperating with us on what we considered a major contribution on the history of influenza in Europe published in "Ecology of Disease." That study also served as the basis for the second chapter of this book and as a topic of interest in Peter Gould's recent contribution, *The Geographer at Work*.

The third phase of effort consisted of publication of some of the works dealing with more recent epidemics of the 1970s and the completion of this book. My thanks go to Gerald J. Karaska for publishing in "Economic Geography" (1984) the only policy-related paper resulting from this project. That paper is the basis for the seventh chapter here. As the various parts of the book were drawn together, analytical aspects of the work clearly reflect the collective influence of Berry, Haggett, Hägerstrand, Brown and Gould, and at the same time, a form of medical geography similar to some of the approaches John Hunter has taken. In fact, John Hunter has followed the project throughout, offering increasing amounts of professional assistance during some of the final and perhaps most critical parts of the synthesis of alternative simulation patterns. Thanks to Hunter's initiative, along with the efforts of Gary Manson, the initial versions of the final simulation findings were first presented to audiences of geographers and health sciences professionals at Michigan State University late in 1984. During this third phase of the project, Paul Lee of Rowman & Littlefield followed progress with the interest of a professional geographer as well as an editor, and I am indebted to Paul for his efforts over the past several years. I look foward to working with Paul Lee and John Hunter in publications on medical geography over the next several years.

This work could not have been completed without other, equally important, forms of assistance. I am quite proud of the graphic materials completed by the Cartographic Laboratory of the University of North Carolina at Charlotte under the direction of Jeff Simpson and Gary Addington. Major typing efforts, at times under different conditions, were accomplished in a very professional manner by Sarah Moore of Midland, NC. While several student assistants helped with the difficult phases of the project, the most meaningful and lengthy support was furnished by Raymond Murray and Pamela Price. Academic environments are such that no book can be completed without the cooperation and assistance of departmental chairs. I will be eternally indebted to Nelson Nunnally for convincing me to make the move from Ohio to North Carolina, and to Alfred Stuart, chairman of the UNCC Department of Geography and Earth Sciences during the several years it took to complete this work.

As always, I am thankful for the support of my family in so many ways. My wife, Carole, will remain an inspiration: she commented on more draft versions of papers and chapters than any other single consultant and/or professional colleague. In the past I thanked our children, Eric and Frances, for golden moments of silence while I was writing. I now thank them for going away to college so that I can continue to write without disruption, but look forward to their homecoming during academic holidays so they can offer "constructive criticisms" to some of my works they may have chanced to encounter within their respective university libraries.

Last, but not least, many thanks to Paul Smith and Steve Jobs.

Preface

As a professional colleague of Gerald Pyle for the past fifteen years in the broad field of medical geography, I am honored to offer some prefatory remarks to this volume. Dr. Pyle, a founding member and first chairperson of the Medical Geography Speciality Group of the Association of American Geographers, through the force of his continuing scholarship occupies the foremost rank among those who endeavor to apply geographic concepts to problems of community diseases and to the delivery of health-care services. His study of cholera in the nineteenth-century United States has become a classic, and other noteworthy research contributions include patterns of heart disease, cancer, and stroke, the spread of measles, spatial and configurations of hospital service areas, and the geography of arbovirus encephalitis.

In the past few years, some selected aspects of Dr. Pyle's research findings on influenza geography have appeared in the serial scientific literature, and now, together with extensive new analyses, they culminate in this capstone volume. Evidence ranges historically from 1580 to 1981 and geographically covers European and North American outbreaks and global pandemics. The focus is the United States. Dramatic highlights include the calamitous pandemic of 1918, the spectacular spread of "Asian flu" of 1957, the ascendency of "Hong Kong flu" in 1968, and the puzzle of "swine flu" in 1976. Pyle's breadth of knowledge allows him to piece together findings from virology and epidemiology and to analyze them in a geographical framework. A rich abundance of figures vividly portray differing spatial patterns of viral diffusions: old and genetically "drifting" viruses, new, abruptly "shifted" viruses, "recycled" infections, endogenous and exogenous outbreaks, endemic "smoldering," multiple epicenters, massive fronts, spring troughs and peaks, "herald" waves and "trailer" waves—altogether a dazzling, illuminating array of maps of viral spread.

In his attempts to develop an effective model of viral spread, Dr. Pyle incorporates the two primary concepts of population mass and distance. He also mathematically invokes central place systems (urban hierarchies), harmonic-wave analysis, and stochastic process. The results are promising. The search continues. The point is the need to incorporate geographic method into strategic planning in public health.

Vitally important in his diffusion research is a goal that Pyle recognizes from the outset: the need to incorporate geographic considerations into official public health strategies to reduce influenza-pneumonia mortality and ultimately to prevent or stifle epidemic outbreaks. Morbidity reduction too, as it affects school and job absenteeism, is a major public health objective. Pyle's findings repeatedly demonstrate the importance of spatial dynamics, not only during pandemics but also in innumerable intervening epidemics, particularly in epicenter formation. As the national debate on vaccination policy proceeds, vexed by questions of indemnity, and as scientific capabilities to monitor viral change increase, with accompanying capacity to manufacture mono- and polyvalent vacines, it becomes increasingly urgent to develop a stronger geographic-spatial methodology in order to improve prediction of rates, directions, and volumes of viral spread, and of the extent, nature, and location of target populations at risk.

Gerald Pyle has produced a landmark volume on the geography of influenza. Typical of any vigorous intellectual exploration, it opens future doors, suggests exciting prospects ahead, and will inspire geographic modeling of this and other diseases. It is a definitive study that, at the same time, persuasively beckons to new horizons in geographic epidemiology.

John M. Hunter
Department of Geography
Department of
   Community Health Science
African Studies Center
Michigan State University

The Diffusion of Influenza

1
Building Bridges in Influenza Geography

Increasing our knowledge of the geography of influenza can be extremely beneficial in disease-prevention programs. The actual disease, often confused with the common cold, is a respiratory infection characterized by headache, fever, and a short dry cough. Usual cases last up to a week, but the disease is especially dangerous to such high-risk groups as the very young and the elderly, as well as those with certain chronic health problems. The elderly, particularly those with overall lower resistance in general, are most susceptible to influenza and its attendant pneumonia complications. Occasionally, there is a neuro-psychological complication known as "post-flu depression" that can last for several weeks or even months. Pneumonia-influenza mortality remains one of the ten leading causes of death in the United States, and it is an even greater threat to human lives in many parts of the Third World.

There are several important reasons why influenza has not been brought under control as well as have many other contagious diseases. Since the disease is caused by a virus, only specific symptoms and second-degree infections can be treated with antibiotics. Immunity can be acquired naturally or induced with a vaccine; however, the appropriate vaccines need to be available at the right times and in the right places. It is also possible for different types of influenza to circulate in different parts of the world at the same time, but often a prevailing strain will periodically become dominant within a region and spread to others over time. Some forms of influenza are more lethal than others, and since the viruses have the ability to go through genetic transformations, resulting in different strains, initial low levels of immunity can often lead to elevated mortality rates. When new forms of influenza surface, they are often either localized or appear in a limited number of relatively proximate epicenters. It is uncommon for similar new forms of influenza to appear simultaneously in locations thousands of miles apart. In addition, there is a tendency to assume automatically that the new forms of the disease originate "someplace else"; hence the labels "Asian flu," "Hong Kong flu," "Russian flu," and the infamous "Spanish Influenza" of 1918. Throughout history, descriptions of influenza epidemics have included accounts of how and when the disease spread from place to place. While many questions may be raised about the accuracy of earlier accounts of influenza diffusion, recent reconstructions of location origins and diffusion pathways have become much clearer.

Still, some aspects of influenza diffusion remain enigmatic. One such characteristic appears to be the actual rate of spread of infection. Contemporary European writers suggest that influenza spread at a "horse pace," and accounts of the 1957 pandemic (worldwide epidemic) followed infected persons across the oceans on ships and overland by bus. However, the 1977–78 influenza epidemic spread through the United States at only about one-tenth the rate of progress of the 1918–19 variant, in spite of vast changes in modes of transportation. Such a comparison is somewhat extreme. The 1918–19 form was the most virulent on record, and virulence does seem to accelerate diffusion. In general, the keys to understanding rates of spread seem to be not only the virulence of an influenza virus but also the balance between immune and susceptible populations. Additional problematic notions include directions of spread and locations of origins of new influenza strains. As summarized by Paul Fine in a 1982 assessment of epidemiological contributions, "Insofar as humans harbor and transmit influenza viruses, one might suppose that these viruses should travel where and when people travel. They should 'go with the people.' But this simple relationship has not been easy to demonstrate."[1] Fine adopted the views of many writing in the 1950s. Before that the disease seems to have spread outward from places of origin in a "directly geographical manner." Given the availability of information on the spatial progress of influenza epidemics, unfortunately acquired only retrospectively, and the geographical scale of analysis, influenza sometimes does appear to radiate outward from specific epicenters. For example, an analysis of the diffusion of influenza in England and Wales in 1957 by Hunter and Young indicated that while the disease initially did radiate outward from several points of early contact, a major diffusion pathway was "toward the people."[2] Clearly, transportation systems serve to expedite the spread of influenza, but population centers serve as magnets and eventually reservoirs for influenza, as well as nodes of connectivity.

Yet another epidemiological puzzle deals with the global origins of influenza pandemics. Since influenza viruses periodically sweep over the surface of the planet, sometimes ignoring transequatorial seasons, it is possible to identify general origins of locations. The best-documented modern event was the pandemic of "Asian flu" of 1957. Almost all the accumulated evidence indicates that the catastrophic event originated in China, and this hypothesis is in keeping with contentions that previous epidemics in other centuries began there also. Since the "China thesis" has gained such justifiable support in the past, there is still a tendency to look to that part of the world first for new influenza strains. The "Hong Kong" strain of influenza first identified in 1968 added even more support to the hypothesis, even though the course of that pandemic is less well documented. There may indeed be something about the natural ecology of south-central Asia that encourages the genetic reconfiguration of influenza viruses, and more research into this possiblility is essential. Nonetheless, this *xenogenic** assumption is so pervasive in the epidemiological literature that it has become a form of dogma. The possibility of "new" or altered forms of influenza first appearing in non-Asian locations cannot be overlooked. Actually, the assumption of exotic origins of diseases, such as syphillis, was well established in Western culture prior to the modern epidemiological era. While the intent of this work is hardly to disavow the above views on the origin and spread of any disease, a detailed examination of the United States experience with major influenza epidemics over the past eighty years in many instances finds the conventional wisdom wanting.

The Influenza Virus and Nomenclature

Almost the first question that must be answered regarding influenza is, "Which kind of virus?" One of the circumstances encountered when examining the literature that has accumulated over the past fifty years is the periodic changes in the nomenclature used to identify virus strains as they are isolated from human and animal sources. Within recent years, extensive and frequent changes in this nomenclature have been necessary to keep up with the accumulation of information about the structure and biological properties of the viron. The current nomenclature reflects the antigenic structure of these viruses, and knowledge of the structure is necessary to understanding the dynamics of movement in human populations.†

The influenza virus is about 80 to 120 nanometers in size.[3] Depicted in Figure 1.1, the core of an influenza viron consists of ribonucleopro-

---

*The term *xenogenic* was recommended by Dr. Jill S. Dubisch, Department of Sociology and Anthropology, The University of North Carolina at Charlotte.

†The following explanation of the virology of influenza was furnished by Dr. Irene T. Schulze, St. Louis University Medical Center, School of Medicine.

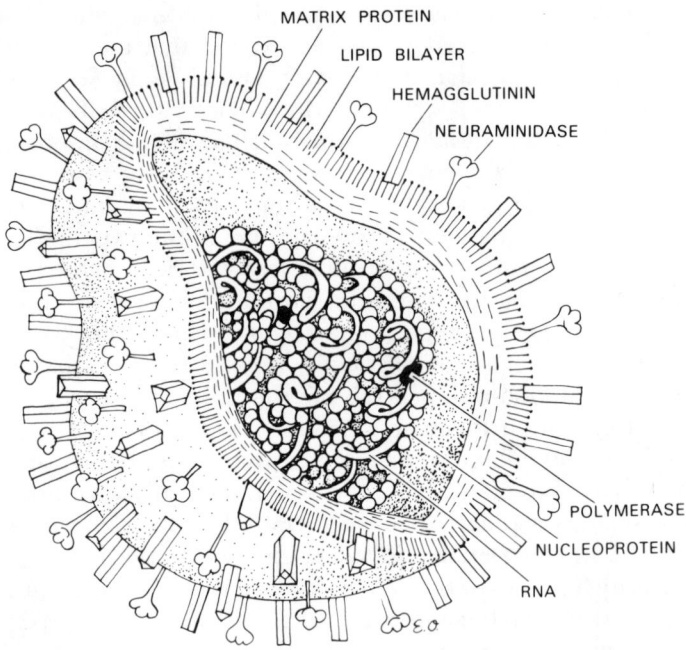

MATRIX PROTEIN
LIPID BILAYER
HEMAGGLUTININ
NEURAMINIDASE
POLYMERASE
NUCLEOPROTEIN
RNA

Figure 1.1. An idealized influenza virus. Note the relationship between the neuraminidase and the hemagglutinin spikes.

tein surrounded by a lipid envelope that contains two types of glycoprotein in the form of spikes. The more numerous of the two are the hemagglutinin spikes responsible for binding the virus to the red cells and host cells. The second type of spike, the neuraminidase, is an enzyme that cleaves termial sialic acid residues from glycoproteins and glycolipids. The neuraminadase facilitates release of progency virus from infected cells as well as the spread of the virus from one cell to another. Antibodies against both the hemagglutinin and neuraminadase may reduce the reproduction of viruses in the host, but only the antibodies against the hemagglutinin neutralize the infectivity of the virus particles.[4]

Different varieties of influenza viruses can now be quickly identified by differences in the ratio of hemagglutinin to neuraminadase spikes. New viral strains do appear periodically. Sometimes minor changes known as "drift" take place,[5] and at others a complete "shift" or major change happens.[6]

Major virus strains are now designated A, B, or C, depending on the antigenic properties of the internal, nonglycosylated component of the viron. Influenza A strains are the most varied of the three types. They have been isolated from animal, avian, and human sources, but B and C strains have thus far been isolated only from humans. The B viruses are less lethal, and they often cause illness within more youthful populations; mortality rates are low.[7] Since the viral hemagglutinins of all influenza B strains contain similar antigenic determinants, they are not divided into subtypes. Less is known about the C strains, but they are apparently not the causes of epidemic illness.

It is now thought that only the A viruses can lead to pandemics, and, depending upon the virulence of the virus, mortality can be extremely high and diffusion rapid. Both forms of genetic change—drift and shift—are influenced by the interrelationship of viruses, host cells, and external as well as internal environments. Clearly, nonimmune humans exposed to recently altered influenza strains have a risk of infection. Infection leads to progressive diffusion of influenza, and surviving hosts acquire immunity to reinfection by the same viral subtype. However, there is no guarantee of immunity to other subtypes. Immunity levels do increase among populations during epidemics, but drift begins to take place, and after immunity levels reach some critical threshold (usually after several years), a major shift can occur and a new dominant A subtype emerges by selection.

Influenza is normally a highly seasonal disease, causing much more illness in the mid-latitudes in winter than in summer. When drift and shift are examined within the context of such seasonality, the interrelationship becomes more clear.[8] As shown in Figure 1.2, a major pandemic can take place when a basically nonimmune population is exposed to a new and virulent virus. Mortality levels are elevated often but not exclusively when external temperatures are lower. Even before, but especially after, a virus has become endemic, annual wintertime peaks may be identified. Meanwhile, minor variations in the form of drift have happened. Thus, a virus introduced as "V2" at one point can gradually drift to "V2$_1$" and then "V2$_2$" over several more influenza seasons. Immunity levels continue to increase, and when a major shift takes place—"V3" in this example—low immunity levels to the new variant can once again result in pandemic influenza. This process does not necessarily repeat itself with predictable regularity, and some pandemics are more deadly than others. Also, while the use of vaccines since the 1940s has substantially reduced mortality rates, the natural processes of drift and shift have not been curtailed. Epidemic outbreaks also tend to be site-specific, thus adding spatial components to shift and drift.

Similar processes take place within nonhuman populations, and strain designations formerly indicated whether influenza A strains were originally isolated from human or animal sources. Accordingly,

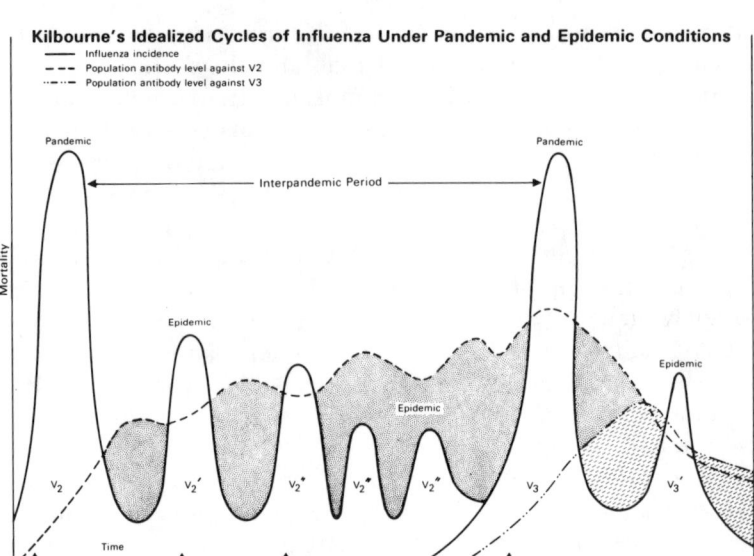

Figure 1.2. The pandemic, epidemic, and interpandemic cycles shown here in idealized form help to explain the relationship between immune and susceptible populations.

reference strains were designated as human, swine, equine, or avian. However, since the hemagglutinin on human and animal isolates can be highly similar in antigenic determinants, the classification and designation of A strains no longer depend on the host from which the virus is isolated. Thus, influenza A viruses from human, avian, and animal sources are placed in the same subtype if they have hemagglutinin antigens in common. Also, since each viral hemagglutinin contains a number of different antigenic determinants, viruses within any one subtype will share some antigenic determinants, but not all of them; therefore, there can be either large or small differences between individual strains within a subtype.

The number of antigenic determinants shared by two strains may be sufficiently high so that antibodies to one strain protect against infections with the other. Conversely, the number of shared determinants may be so low that no crossprotection is observed. Thus, viruses isolated from the human population in consecutive waves of an epidemic may be crossprotective because they are highly similar antigenically, whereas strains ten years apart may have few antigens in common and afford no crossprotection. The latter situation in 1947 led to the conclusion at the time that a new subtype of influenza A had appeared in the human population (Chapter 4). Neither previous influenza illness nor vaccination protected individuals from

Table 1.1 Subtypes of Hemagglutinin Antigens of Influenza A Viruses

Subtypes	Previous Subtypes (1971 system)
H1	H0, H1, Hsw1
H2	H2
H3	H3, Heq2, Hav7
H4	Hav4
H5	Hav5
H6	Hav6
H7	Heq1, Hav1
H8	Hav8
H9	Hav9
H10	Hav2
H11	Hav3
H12	Hav10

the influenza A virus strain that appeared that year. Retrospective analysis has shown, however, that both the original A strains and the 1947 isolates (designated A′ at the time they were isolated) do indeed contain common antigens. These viruses, along with animal isolates with common antigens, such as the swine influenza isolated in 1931 (Chapter 3), are now designated H1 (see Table 1.1). The second virus glycoprotein, the neuraminidase also exists in different antigenic forms. Again, strains are grouped into subtypes based on the presence and absence of common antigens. There are nine neuraminidase subtypes among the influenza A viruses (see Table 1.2).

This system of nomenclature was adopted by the World Health Organization in 1980 and is currently in use throughout the world.

Table 1.2 Subtypes of Neuraminidase Antigens of Influenza A Viruses

Subtypes	Previous Subtypes (1971 system)
N1	N1
N2	N2
N3	Nav2, Nav3
N4	Nav4
N5	Nav5
N6	Nav1
N7	Neq1
N8	Neq2
N9	Nav6

Source: Centers for Disease Control, *Morbidity and Mortality Weekly Report* 79, no. 42 (October 24, 1980), p. 515.

Strains are further identified by place, isolate number (when known), and year of isolation. Thus, in 1957 a virus strain with internal nonglycosylated components that crossreacted with previous A strains was isolated in Singapore (Chapter 5). The hemagglutinin of that virus contained none of the antigenic determinants found in H1 strains. Its neuraminidase was also completely different in antigenic determinants from N1 strains. This virus strain is now designated A/Singapore/57 (H2N2). All influenza A virus strains isolated from 1957 until 1968 were found to have antigenic determinants on both the neuraminidase and hemagglutinin that crossreacted with the 1957 strain; these are all H2N2 strains. The viruses identified in the late 1960s (such as A/Hong Kong/68) are designated H3N2 (Chapter 6) because they contain a different hemagglutinin (H3) and a crossreacting neuraminidase (N2).

Thus far, human influenza viruses that cause widespread disease have been found to contain hemagglutinin subtypes H1, H2, or H3 and neuraminidase subtypes N1 or N2. As these viruses are transmitted from individual to individual in the human population, mutations occur in both the hemagglutinin and neuraminidase genes. Such mutations can bring about differences in the antigenic properties of these two viral proteins. Although strains isolated close together in time are likely to be similar in antigenic determinants, this is not always the case. For example, in 1977 an H1N1 virus was isolated in Russia and was subsequently found in various countries, including the United States (Chapter 7). This virus, A/USSR/77(H1N1), is much more closely related to a virus strain isolated in Fort Warren, New Jersey, in 1950 (A/FW/1/50[H1N1]) than to the H1N1 strains isolated at Fort Dix in 1976. Thus, proximity in place and time of isolation is not necessarily an indication of the antigenic relatedness of individual isolates.

Currently, the strain designations indicate the type of internal antigens (A, B, or C) and, with influenza A strains, the types of hemagglutinin (H1–12) and neuraminidase (N1–N9). They also indicate the time and place of isolation, but not the degree of similarity between strains within a subtype.

Influenza Surveillance Methods

The cyclical nature of influenza pandemics and epidemics, the ability of the disease to diffuse rapidly from epicenters, and long-term experiences with national or regional monitoring of the spatial progression or morbidity and mortality reporting have all resulted in international and national surveillance systems. As would be expected, the accuracy and range of geographical coverage varies considerably from one country to another. In the United States there has been national surveillance of temporal aspects of influenza-related mortality for most of this century, but geographical coverage has varied in accordance with urban growth and change, federal perceptions of the severity of the problem, and Public Health Service policy decisions. With the exception of a gap of several years during the 1950s, there has been weekly public reporting of influenza-pneumonia mortality from key urban centers since the autumn of 1918. Deaths from influenza with pneumonia complications have been used as a statistically verifiable measure of the magnitude of the disease problem, because influenza-morbidity reporting is usually incomplete, particularly during nonepidemic periods. Increased influenza-morbidity reporting generally is an indication that an epidemic is already well established. Thus, for purposes of maintaining surveillance systems, the United States and many other countries use pneumonia-influenza, or P&I, mortality reporting on a regular (usually weekly) basis as a measure of the severity of the disease.

Today, if P&I mortality accounts for 4.5 percent or more of the total deaths reported within the United States during any given week, especially during the early autumn, there is a high probability that an influenza epidemic is underway. The inherent weakness in using national totals is that the figures represent a sort of average and do not always account for localized early influenza-diffusion epicenter formation. One example of this phenomenon was the 1976 influenza outbreak in Philadelphia (see Chapter 7). Also, in spite of temporal lags between influenza morbidity and P&I mortality reporting, the latter measure, when observed on a place-by-place comparative basis, does represent the best available measure for determining diffusion patterns of the disease.

In addition to the weekly P&I reporting, the United States surveillance system functions with linkages to the World Health Organization network. If a new influenza virus is isolated in another part of the world and it begins to spread geographically, public health alerts can be issued. In such a manner, morbidity reports are used as warnings of possible mortality, and vaccines, if available, can be distributed. Such would be the ideal situation and the rationale for continuously improving surveillance systems. The system has grown over time, and two of the most significant improvements were, unfortunately, prompted by influenza pandemics. Prior to the devastating 1918–19 pandemic (see Chapter 3), influenza-mortality reporting was limited to national totals on a weekly basis. While the disease was one of the leading causes of death, it was not perceived to be a major health threat until thousands died within a matter of weeks. Still, the Public

Health Service responded promptly, given the status of data processing at that time, and within a month of the pandemic onset a weekly
influenza reporting system that was to last for decades was put into
effect.

None of the influenza epidemics in the 1920s, 1930s, and 1940s
came close to the tragedy of 1918. As improved medical treatments
for secondary bacterial infections were introduced and vaccines were
developed, the overall incidence of P&I mortality decreased substantially. This trend, along with the magnitude of the influenza problem
in 1918, is shown in Figure 1.3. No doubt as a result of this downward
trend, the Public Health Service made a decision to curtail the weekly
reporting of P&I mortality in the mid-1950s. The system was reini-
tiated, however, after the arrival of a new strain of influenza (H2N2)
in 1957. The worldwide surveillance system had functioned during
the H2N2 pandemic, and the arrival of the strain in the United States
during the summer of 1957 was expected; however, spatial patterns
of diffusion could not be adequately anticipated because of the lack of
urban-based weekly P&I mortality reporting. When the weekly re-

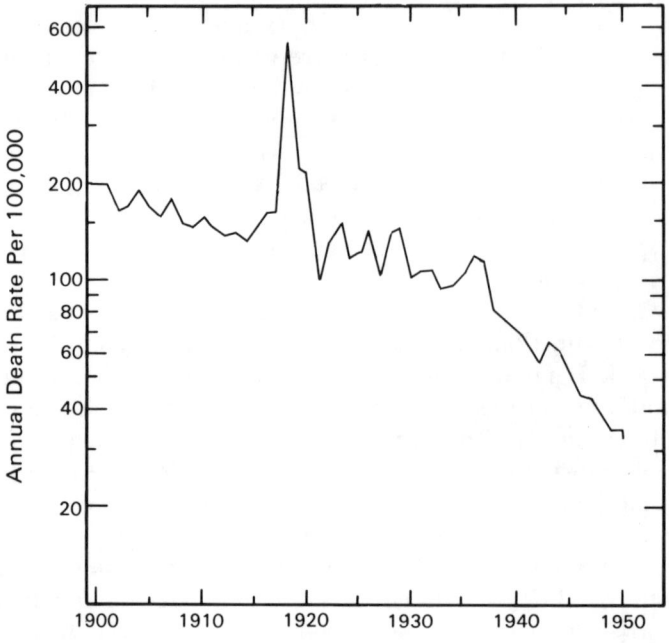

Trends in P & I Mortality, 1900-1950

Figure 1.3. The long-term declines in Influenza-Pneumonia (P&I) mortality in the United States are shown here
interrupted by epidemics and the 1918–20 pandemic.

porting system was eventually restored, improvements were also made regarding methods of data analysis.

Refinements in methods of temporal analysis were made so that unusual increases in influenza activity could be recognized more quickly. The methods that had been used between the two pandemics were developed by Selwyn Collins and his colleagues at the Public Health Service, and they now serve as an excellent historical account of past influenza activity (Chapters 3 and 4). As a form of measurement, Collins used a "normal" seasonal curve based on the several previous years to identify any aberrations in expected trends. This method was considered inadequate when weekly urban reporting was revitalized in the late 1950s, primarily because Collins had used crude mortality rates. After influenza surveillance was deemed to be the responsibility of the Communicable Disease Center (now the Centers for Disease Control), a statistical method developed by Robert Serfling was adopted to reduce the risk of failure to recognize an epidemic.[9] The Serfling method differed from that of Collins in at least two major ways: (1) the total number of deaths was presumed to be a better measure of the influenza problem than crude rates; and (2) a least-squares regression based on any previous five-years' experience was used to estimate "expected" mortality. If the number of influenza-related deaths reported exceeded the anticipated threshold, there was "excess" mortality and probably an epidemic, as was the case in 1968 (Chapter 6).

The Serfling model is curvilinear, fitting a sine/cosine curve (Fig. 1.4) in the estimation of epidemic thresholds for a given influenza season. One of the first applications of this method was the determination of the magnitude of the H2N2 pandemic in the United States (Chapter 5). Serfling was able to identify two distinct epidemic waves in this manner. The method was used by the United States Public Health Service for more than twenty-five years and adopted in other countries. The technique was further refined by Houseworth and Langmuir in the 1970s[10] and used in conjunction with an alternative approach to monitoring in the early 1980s. The alternative procedure, as put forth by Choi and Thacker, uses a Box-Jenkins (ARIMA) model, with P&I deaths as a proportion of all mortality during any given week.[11] In spite of continued refinements in surveillance of the disease, neither method "predicted" the epidemic of 1980–81 (Chapter 8). That circumstance had less to do with statistical methods used than with geographical scale of analysis. Again, when only national or major regional P&I data are used, the early impact of an epidemic can be masked. This condition appears to be particularly important when an epidemic is not of extraneous origin.

Since influenza data are available for many reporting cities during

**Modifications of the Serfling
Model: Early 1980 s**

$$Y= \quad a \; + \; \beta_1 t \; + \; \beta_2 \cos\left(\frac{2\pi t}{52}\right) + \; \beta_3 \sin\left(\frac{2\pi t}{52}\right) + \; \beta_4 \cos\left(\frac{2\pi t}{26}\right) + \; \beta_5 \sin\left(\frac{2\pi t}{26}\right) + \; E$$

$$Y= \quad \binom{\text{average}}{\text{mortality}} + \;\; \text{(trend)} + \quad \text{(52 week cycle)} \quad + \qquad \text{(26 week cycle)} \; + \; E$$

Where   Y = estimated number of deaths

a = constant

t = time interval

E = random error

$$\beta\cos\varphi + \;\beta\sin\varphi = C_1 \cos(\varphi - \theta)$$

Where C_1 = amplitude

φ = frequency

θ = phase angle

Figure 1.4. Serfling's model, developed after the H2N2 pandemic, was modified several times over twenty-five years, but it was still basically a regression technique intended to estimate levels of influenza activity.

various epidemics in the United States, it seems logical that such information can be used in the reconstruction of past patterns of diffusion in greater geographical detail than previously attempted. Such reconstructions have in fact been accomplished in this work, but the final results do not necessarily reflect the many earlier, erroneous assumptions and repeated trials that subsequently added a better understanding of some of the problems no doubt encountered by Collins, Serfling, Langmuir, and others, who may have attempted to use individual urban P&I reporting data over extended periods. The first consideration in dealing with such information is that just as the relative importance of a given city varies over time within the national urban system, so does the quality and availability of reporting resources. As the country became increasingly urban during this century, the number of cities reporting has changed over time; some with accelerated growth rates have been added to the sample, and others that have declined no longer report influenza deaths. Today, 121 cities are listed in the Centers for Disease Control (CDC) weekly reports of P&I mortality, but only 95 are providing meaningful data as determined by simple confidence tests. These cities make up a sample of approximately 25 percent of the United States population, a large enough proportion to be statistically useful.

Repeated experimentation with crude mortality rates, numbers of deaths, and influenza-to-total ratios by city have revealed that all of these measures, sometimes used in combination, help us to understand influenza diffusion. The criticisms of Collins's earlier use of rates are valid in that such a measure is a form of "overcontrol" that can fail to identify an epidemic. In some instances, large urban places like New York City may have a lower influenza death rate than the national average but a higher number of deaths than any other city. Conversely, a smaller city may have a high rate and fewer actual deaths. This problem can be resolved by examining a sufficient number of adjacent cities, and if enough have a higher-than-average rate, an influenza outbreak is apparent. In addition, it is sometimes necessary to use rates in statistical tests to counteract statistical problems that arise when numbers of deaths are used in geographical analysis. The distance-decay formulations in Chapter 7 help us to identify the direction and rate of influenza diffusion. It is also important in such studies to understand the numerical magnitude of the problem. Significant numbers of deaths in cities with overall low rates do not mean that mortality remains low as the disease spreads within cities and surrounding areas. The maps of progressively increasing numbers of cases in subsequent chapters are instructive in reconstructing the temporal spread of influenza epidemics. While it might be assumed that such a procedure would normally be an indication only of the hierarchical nature of the urban system, this is not always the case, as was particularly true during the late 1960s (Chapter 6). The basis for Serfling's use of numbers of influenza deaths in temporal models continues to be important in geographical studies because it is the best measure of the actual magnitude of the problem.

Ratio-scale comparisons are also essential in understanding the time-series nature of influenza cycles. Since influenza is essentially a "wintertime" disease, with far fewer deaths reported during the summer, the proportion of influenza mortality in relation to all other causes is usually far greater during colder temperature periods. As a result, using a proportional scale with influenza reporting data over a period of several years reflects seasonal oscillations of the disease in a manner that is similar to the Serfling method. Expected mortality can be determined on the basis of the past several seasons. Under epidemic conditions, actual mortality can exceed what is expected early in the autumn and sometimes in the late summer. Using the ratio method, epidemic conditions exist when more than 4.5 percent of all deaths for a sustained period, such as four to six weeks, are caused by influenza. The epidemic may be part of a worldwide pandemic of a new strain, or it might also be an unusual flare-up of a prevailing type of influenza. This ratio must be monitored in more geographical detail than at major national or regional levels in order to identify several characteristic phenomena. The most apparent comparative oscillation often noted is that "lead" and "lag" cities stand out (Fig. 1.5). While some places approximate the national average with respect to summer lulls followed by increases in the autumn, individual and often geographical clusters of cities emerge as lead locations, sometimes a month or so ahead of others. For some reason, other cities lag. Some of these differences are due to the variable intensity of viral activity the previous spring, but the overall result is that influenza reporting from some cities is on the decline at the same time it is on the increase in others.

Today, insufficient information is available to determine if major differences exist in the types of viruses causing the variable numbers of influenza deaths. When a new strain is introduced into the population, however, it is most likely to be isolated within the lead places because of probable overall lower immunity levels. A similar circumstance could arise after a certain amount of viral drift. Given these

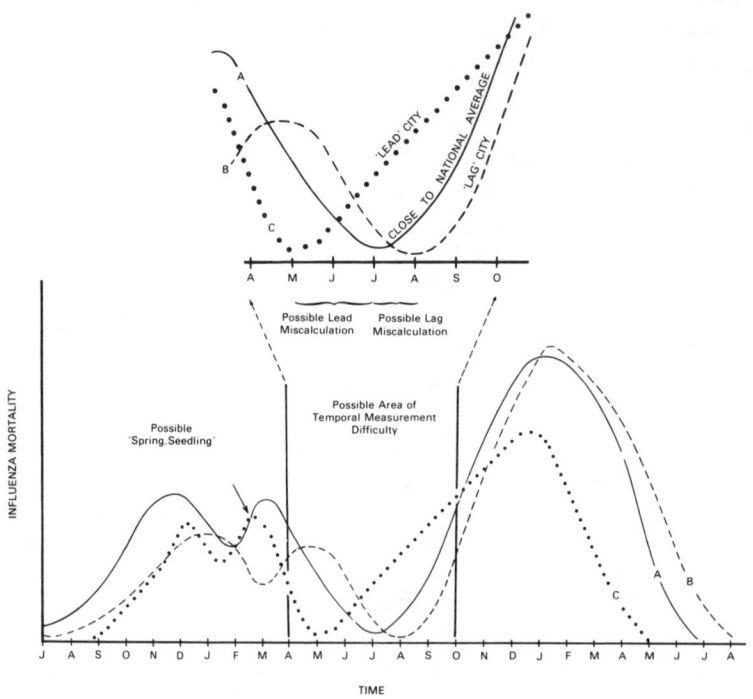

Figure 1.5. One area of measurement difficulty consists of possible increases in influenza activity due to the arrival of a new virus in one city while a prevailing strain is still on the decline.

conditions, the best method of identifying sustained increases is to monitor the number of cases reported in the lead places, with particular attention given to specific locations that have exceeded the epidemic-threshold ratio. When these relative differences are mapped (see Chapters 7 and 8), diffusion epicenters can be identified. In addition, temporal peaks in epidemic waves can be further identified, although in a more retrospective but nonetheless useful fashion, by indicating the fiftieth percentiles of the various numerical distributions. These two measures used in conjunction are of enormous assistance in replicating actual patterns of diffusion. The key to this procedure is to know when influenza is definitely on the increase.

Actual times of late summer/early autumn increase are often difficult to determine because of periodic limited summer flare-ups in influenza deaths and more extensive late winter/early spring outbreaks. The former are more localized, but the latter sometimes reach regional miniepidemic proportions after wintertime peaks have been reached. Conversely, some of the springtime peaks identified in this study may simply be late seasonal outbreaks signifying delayed main waves. At any rate, such phenomena often result in delayed autumn increases, particularly if the same strain of virus prevails. One of the most perplexing of the phenomena that emerge in the examination of some of the major epidemics of influenza in this century is that most were preceded by spring outbreaks. In some instances the spring outbreaks have been definitely attributed to strains of influenza that had prevailed for a decade or more, only to be followed several months later by epidemics caused by a shifted strain. This was apparently the case in 1957 (Chapter 5), 1968 (Chapter 6), and possibly in the late 1970s (Chapter 7).

The great pandemic of 1918 was also preceded by unusually high reporting of influenza during the spring, but not nearly of the intensity of what occurred during the autumn. There have also been instances of "spring peaking" followed by wintertime epidemics that seem to have been caused by the same or a closely related strain; for example, during the influenza seasons of 1928–29 (Chapter 3) and 1943–44 (Chapter 4). This phenomenon has been frequent enough to suggest that some form of "seeding" mentioned periodically by influenza researchers may be taking place. Geographically, the meaning of spring seeding is somewhat elusive, because influenza epicenters often form in the autumn in locations quite distant from places characterized by the earlier outbreaks. In the context of general influenza surveillance, the springtime phenomenon can be used as an early-warning indicator of a pending epidemic, but it apparently cannot be used reliably to determine specific major outbreak locations within the simulation-modeling process.

Theoretical Considerations in Simulating Influenza Diffusion

The theoretical foundations for constructing the influenza-simulation procedures posited in Chapter 8 have been derived first from the development of an understanding of the disease agent and how illness data are acquired and then from methodological contributions of historians, epidemiologists, and geographers. The historical foundation is important because the reconstruction of past epidemic patterns offers clues to probable locations of origins, as well as variable patterns and rates of diffusion during different pandemic episodes. Beginning with the contributions of Beveridge,[12] Crosby,[13] and Patterson[14] as past specific accounts of the diffusion of influenza, methods of the medical historian were further used to develop the expositions of the spread of the disease in Chapters 2 and 3. These findings indicate, as with other diseases, that there were general perceptions of how influenza might spread over time and geographic space prior to the discovery of the specific agent responsible. While some earlier notions of the disease are not supported by scientific fact, others have continued to influence modern-day epidemiology, such as the "China thesis." Perhaps more important, however, the historical reconstructions indicate that a typology of diffusion patterns, ranging from multiple epicenter outbreaks to massive frontal movements, has operated perhaps for centuries.

The epidemiological foundations of influenza geography are important inputs in simulating the disease. For example, the several time-series methods already discussed formed the basis for the harmonic analysis in the "repeated events" simulation alternative in Chapter 8. In addition to such aspects as the nature of available influenza information and how it can be calibrated over spans of time, there are many important explanations of the "neighborhood effects" of the disease. For example, it has been demonstrated with limited (less than national or regional) samples that, with little or no immunity, the geographical spread of the disease is mathematically geometrical. With high immunity levels, the rate of spread is mathematically and geographically more linear. Clearly, a wide range of possibilities exists between these extremes, and epidemiologists have suggested the transfer of infection between individuals because of undirected subclinical cases at one end of the spectrum and the possibility of some individuals operating as "superspreaders" at the other.

Many community-based influenza geographies have been accomplished by epidemiologists, and they assist in understanding some of the macroscale patterns contained in this book. There is a scale gap in the transition from community to national levels. For example, the models developed by Elveback and her colleagues to replicate the

H2N2 and H3N2 epidemics are restricted to communities of approximately 1,000 persons.[15] Bailey has indicated that it is less difficult to model measles epidemics (also cyclical), and problems arise when attempting to use existing epidemiological models to explain influenza epidemics in populations above 250,000.[16] The basic reason for these conditions is that most of the epidemiological models are concerned with the identification of index cases, and limited numbers of infected individuals often serve as the basis for predicting major consecutive epidemic waves.

Two recent departures from previous trends can be found in the works of Soviet and British influenza researchers. Working with large-population influenza-diffusion models, a group of Soviet researchers has been using daily morbidity reports from 100 large urban areas with 100,000 persons or more since the 1960s. Their models have incorporated numbers of cases, susceptibles, the duration of cases, overall population, a migration factor that resembles a partial gravity model, and a somewhat elusive "transmission factor" that is invariant from one place to another in most empirical tests.[17] This results in a procedure using continuous data, with infections predicted on the basis of the average number of cases that can be spread by a single person. According to the Soviet researchers, the results of predictions match actual diffusion patterns. Applying the models developed by the Soviet researchers to discrete, weekly mortality data from England and Wales, Spicer found that most of the procedures used tended to overpredict the onset of influenza in the autumn and indicate springtime declines before they actually took place.[18] These efforts indicate that epidemiologists are becoming more concerned with how influenza epidemics might be expected to spread, but most major efforts in the United States still have been directed toward either defining national epidemic thresholds numerically or attempting to determine how the disease spreads within small communitites. To close this scale gap it is necessary to apply some of the methods developed by geographers to the study of influenza diffusion.

The contributions of geographers take two forms: (1) analyses of the spatial diffusion of specific diseases and (2) studies in the diffusion of innovation. Most disease-diffusion studies have been done by medical geographers, and they range in scale from municipal to continental coverage. For example, the examination of spread pathways during several nineteenth-century cholera epidemics in the United States revealed that as cities continued to grow and develop, the hierarchical nature of the urban system became increasingly important as a determinant factor in disease diffusion.[19] Separate spatial analyses of the diffusion of cholera in Africa in the 1970s by

Stock and Kwofie led to additional general principles of the diffusion of that disease. Stock concluded that cholera-diffusion patterns can take four forms: coastal, linear, hierarchical, and radial. He further suggested that different combinations of these forms can operate simultaneously, depending upon the regional settlement system.[20] Kwofie used polynomial trend-surface analysis to show the spread of cholera in West Africa during primary, saturation, and waning phases.[21]

In a more recent study, Adesina demonstrated that cholera diffused in the city of Ibadan in a distance-decay fashion outward from points of origin.[22] McGlashan discovered similar distance-decay mechanisms operating in Tasmania when he examined the diffusion of viral hepatitis.[23] He showed how the disease spread from urban places in discrete diffusion zones in a general radial-hierarchical fashion, lending additional support to the findings of other medical geographers. In a more comprehensive analysis of the diffusion of hepatitis in the Wollongona district of New South Wales between 1954 and 1970, Brownlea demonstrated mathematically that the disease has the ability to spread at a rate faster and slower than random.[24] Brownlea identified "ecological pathways" leading into "clinical fronts," and he developed a predictive model that approximated the actual situation. One of the few medical geographers attempting to test the general theories of spatial diffusion put forth by Hägerstrand with disease data, Brownlea found that settlement size and distance-decay formulations are necessary ingredients in such model building.

The second category of diffusion studies by geographers has been largely built upon some of the premises, as modified over more than thirty years, of Hägerstrand's seminal works on the diffusion of innovation. Hägerstrand put forth some basic principles on the process of adoption of innovation supported by empirical tests that subsequently led to numerous scientific applications by geographers.[25] Many of these related analyses, recently synthesized by Brown,[26] have stressed the importance of settlement size and distance-decay mechanisms and how they influence hierarchical and contagious diffusion. Berry has shown how such models can be calibrated within an actual temporal context,[27] and Brown and his colleagues have offered numerous empirical applications of diffusion theories.[28] As explained by Gould,[29] cones of resolution representing distance-decay effects can be fit to centers of innovation in the form of what Hägerstrand termed a Mean Information Field (MIF), consisting of cells with outwardly decreasing probabilities of acceptance. By defining time in discrete units, the MIF can be moved about over a larger geographical area through a random-selection process. Thus, with a hierarchically based premise of spatial diffusion, cones of resolution would continue to grow about settlements in accordance with city size because it is assumed that larger places would tend to adopt innovations first. This approach, along with several others, is applied to the simulation of influenza diffusion in more detail in Chapter 8. Other, related studies of spatial diffusion that have implications to modeling the spread of influenza include Morrill's simulation of ghetto expansion in Seattle,[30] Haggett's modeling of measles diffusion,[31] and the recent comprehensive analysis of measles in Iceland by Cliff et al.[32]

While most of these theoretical approaches are considered in the alternative influenza-simulation models in Chapter 8, the attributes of different strains of influenza and how they may have spread geographically during past epidemics require examination first. Also, this is essentially not a policy-oriented work, but because influenza has taken so many lives over the years, an examination of attitudes about national inoculation programs cannot be ignored. For this reason, the policy evaluations in Chapter 5, 6, and 7 have been included, and with the final recommendations they also address the geography of influenza-inoculation policy in the United States. Neither is this study simply a simulation exercise. Instead, the intent is to suggest alternative future influenza-diffusion patterns so that geographical strategies can become a major part of any control and prevention program.

Notes

1. Paul Fine, "Applications of Mathematical Models to the Epidemiology of Influenza: A Critique," in Philip Selby, ed., *Influenza Models: Prospects for Development and Use* (Lancaster, Boston, and The Hague: MTP Press, 1982), pp. 505–53.
2. John M. Hunter and Jonathan C. Young, "Diffusion of Influenza in England and Wales," *Annals, Association of American Georgraphers* 61 (December 1971), pp. 637–53.
3. Martin M. Kaplan and Robert G. Webster, "The Epidemiology of Influenza," *Scientific American* 273 (1977), pp. 88–106.
4. N. G. Wrigley, "Electron Microscopy of Influenza Virus," *British Medical Bulletin* 35 (1979), pp. 35–38.
5. G. C. Schild et al., "Antigenic Variation of Current Type A Influenza Viruses: Antigenic Characteristics of the Variants and Their Geographic Distribution," *Bulletin, World Health Organization* 48 (1973), pp. 269–78.
6. Charles Stuart-Harris, "The Influenza Problem," *Medical Laboratory Technology* 32 (1975), pp. 161–69.
7. P. Palese and J. F. Young, "Variation of Influenza A, B and C Viruses," *Science* 115 (1982), p. 1468.
8. Edwin D. Kilbourne, "The Influenza Viruses and Influenza—An Introduction," in Edwin D. Kilbourne, ed., *The Influenza Viruses and Influenza* (New York: Academic Press, 1975).
9. Robert E. Serfling, "Methods for Current Statistical Analysis of Excess Pneumonia-Influenza Deaths," *Public Health Reports* 78 (1963), pp. 494–506.
10. Jere Housworth and Alexander D. Langmuir, "Excess Mortality from Epidemic Influenza, 1957–1966," *American Journal of Epidemiology* 100 (1974), pp. 40–48.

11. K. Choi and S. B. Thacker, "An Evaluation of Influenza Mortality Surveillance, 1962–1979. II: Percentage of Pneumonia and Influenza Deaths as an Indicator of Influenza Activity," *American Journal of Epidemiology* 113 (1981), pp. 227–30.
12. W. I. B. Beveridge, *Influenza: The Last Great Plague: An Unfinished Story of Discovery* (New York: Prodist, 1977).
13. Alfred W. Crosby, Jr., *Epidemic and Peace, 1918* (Westport, Conn.: Greenwood Press, 1976).
14. K. David Patterson, "The Demographic Impact of the 1918–19 Influenza Pandemic in Sub-Saharan Africa: A Preliminary Assessment," in Christopher Fyfe and David McMaster, eds., *African Historical Demography*, vol. 2 (Edinburgh: University of Edinburgh, 1981), pp. 401–31.
15. L. R. Elveback et al., "An Influenza Simulation Model for Immunization Studies," *American Journal of Epidemiology* 103 (1976), pp. 152–65.
16. N. T. J. Bailey, *The Mathematical Theory of Infectious Diseases and Its Applications* (London: Charles Griffith and Company, 1975).
17. O. V. Baroyan et al., "Computer Modeling of Influenza Epidemics for the Whole Country (USSR)," *Advances in Applied Probability* 3 (1971), pp. 224–446.
18. Clive C. Spicer, "The Mathematical Modeling of Influenza Epidemics," *British Medical Bulletin* 35 (1979), pp. 23–28.
19. G. F. Pyle, "The Diffusion of Cholera in the United States in the Nineteenth Century," *Geographical Analysis* 1 (1969), pp. 59–75.
20. R. Stock, *Cholera in Africa* (London: International African Institute, 1976).
21. Kwame Mayer Kwofie, "A Spatio-Temporal Analysis of Cholera Diffusion in Western Africa," *Economic Georgraphy* (52) (1976), pp. 127–35.
22. H. O. Adesina, "The Diffusion of Cholera Outside Ibadan City, Nigeria, 1971," *Social Science and Medicine* 18 (1984), pp. 421–28.
23. Neil D. McGlashan, "Viral Hepatitis in Tasmania," *Social Science and Medicine* 110 (1977), pp. 731–44.
24. A. A. Brownlea, "An Urban Ecology of Infectious Disease: City of Greater Wollongong, Shell Harbour," *Australian Geographer* 10 (1967), pp. 169–87.
25. Torsten Hägerstrand, *The Propagation of Innovation Waves*. Lund Studies in Geography, series B, no. 4 (Gleerup, Sweden: June 1952).
26. Lawrence A. Brown, *Innovation Diffusion: A New Perspective* (New York and London: Methuen, 1981).
27. Brian J. L. Berry, "Hierarchical Diffusion: The Basis of Developmental Filtering and Spread in a System of Growth Centers," in N. M. Hansen, ed., *Growth Centers in Regional Economic Development* (New York: The Free Press, 1972), and *Growth Centers in the American Urban System* (Cambridge: Ballinger, 1973).
28. Lawrence A. Brown and Kevin R. Cox, "Empirical Regularities in the Diffusion of Innovation," *Annals, Association of American Geographers* 61 (1971), pp. 551–59.
    Lawrence A. Brown, et al., "The Diffusion of Cable Television in Ohio: A Case Study of Diffusion Agency Location Patterns and Processes of the Polynuclear Type," *Economic Georgraphy* 50 (1974), pp. 285–99.
    Lawrence A. Brown and S. G. Philliber, "The Diffusion of a Population-Related Innovation: The Planned Parenthood Affiliate," *Social Science Quarterly* 58 (1977), pp. 215–27.
29. Peter P. Gould, *Spatial Diffusion*, Resource Paper Series, no. 4 (Washington, D.C.: Association of American Geographers, 1969).
30. Richard M. Morrill, "The Negro Ghetto: Problems and Alternatives," *The Geographical Review* 55 (1965), pp. 339–61.
31. Peter Haggett, "Hybridizing Alternative Models of an Epidemic Diffusion Process," *Economic Geography* 52 (1976), pp. 136–46.
32. A. D. Cliff et al., *Spatial Diffusion: An Historical Geography of Epidemics in an Island Community* (Cambridge: Cambridge University Press, 1981).

2

Precursors to the Conventional Wisdom: Some Earlier European Experiences

Historical accounts of influenza epidemics include descriptions of geographical diffusion pathways, and many epidemiological studies since the 1950s still reflect a conventional wisdom about influenza geography based on what appears to have happened centuries earlier.[1] The most commonly held belief is that influenza pandemics have their origins in China or central Asia, and when new strains emerge for a variety of biological reasons, explosions of the disease occur and it pours outward as would an army of savage Tatars. Of course, we tend to have a clearer memory of the most severe pandemics, and in many countries historical accounts of other important events were placed within time frames based on what happened before and after major pandemics. Certainly this was true of the Black Death of the fourteenth century, and it might also have been true in parts of Europe (as it is in some West African villages) during the pandemic of 1918–19 had it not been for the casualties of World War I. Still, the somewhat mysterious pandemic of 1918–19 took an extremely heavy toll of 20 to 40 million lives,[2] and that episode serves as a comparative pivotal point in chronicles of the disease.

Even in the 1980s there is some speculation as to whether the pandemic, once commonly referred to as Spanish Influenza, was caused by what is now known as the swine flu virus.[3] Some researchers are of the opinion that the 1918–19 pandemic also began in China, but others believe that it started in the United States in milder form during the spring of 1918, underwent some change in genetic composition, and subsequently ravaged the entire planet from Europe.[4] Regardless where it began, the xenogenic assumption continued to prevail in epidemiological studies.[5] Theories of extraneous origins of

---

This chapter was adapted from earlier research conducted with Dr. K. David Patterson, Department of History, University of North Carolina at Charlotte. (See Note 5.)

influenza epidemics and pandemics have dominated European accounts of influenza diffusion for centuries, and China has remained the culprit in a multitude of twentieth-century studies on the origins of influenza pandemics.

This chapter will examine the historical geography of influenza in Europe prior to the 1918–19 pandemic and illustrate the development of beliefs about the geographical origins of influenza in Western society. Several medical aspects of the disease should be kept in mind. The first set of epidemiological attributes are those pertaining to the cyclical nature of the disease because of the balance between immunes and susceptibles mentioned within Chapter 1. It should also be remembered that influenza outbreaks are frequently followed by second and sometimes third waves of illness and death.[6] In addition, wintertime influenza peaks are usually the most severe, but pandemic waves often begin in the late summer or early fall.[7] Influenza pandemics and epidemics are often preceded by springtime herald waves of illness in locations peripheral to outbreak epicenters,[8] and it is most common during an influenza epidemic for mortality rates to be highest among the very young and elderly, but notable exceptions include particularly virulent viruses attacking those twenty to forty years of age.[9] While it is theoretically possible for there to be an infinite number of influenza viral forms, a relatively few such types have apparently reappeared or recycled historically.[10] These and other epidemic aspects of influenza emerge periodically in historical descriptions of the diffusion of the disease in Europe.

In this chapter, influenza-diffusion pathways are also examined with reference to contemporary trade and transportation systems, political alliances, and important historical events, thus helping to explain why the disease seems to have spread in certain directions. The European experience is a logical place to start because information is available to reconstruct influenza diffusion over several centuries, and Europe was the first continent to develop more modern systems of cities and the transportation networks that linked them. Furthermore, narratives in several languages offer valuable cultural perceptions of the disease and how it might have spread. An equally important reason for examining the diffusion of influenza in Europe first is that views of the disease that originated there have also diffused to North America and other parts of the world.

Given current knowledge, it is assumed in the following reconstructions that the pandemics or epidemics were caused by different types of influenza A. Evidence at least suggests forms of viral recycling prior to the 1918–19 pandemic, as well as later during the twentieth century. If there is any strongly similar circumstance, it appears to be the relationship between the "Asian" influenza of 1957 and the pandemic of 1889–92. During the late 1950s, serologic testing of elderly persons who were known not to have had influenza recently indicated previously acquired immunity, thus giving rise to the hypothesis that the more recent strain had circulated before. More recent evidence on the recurrence of viruses over long periods reinforces the hypothesis that a limited number of viral strains have circulated periodically in the past and will continue to do so in the future.[11]

Some Major European Pandemics

People have probably suffered from influenza for thousands of years. Viruses identical or closely related to human pathogens infect ducks, turkeys, swine, horses, and other warm-blooded vertebrates,[12] and man probably acquired influenza when he first domesticated animals. The development of agriculture and the rise of towns provided sufficient numbers of potential hosts to sustain epidemics. Influenza or a similar disease is mentioned in fifth-century B.C. writings ascribed to Hippocrates and by chroniclers throughout the Middle Ages. Such scholars as Hirsch (1882)[13] and Finkler (1898) tabulated apparent outbreaks from the twelfth century,[14] but these early epidemics are not adequately documented, and clinical descriptions are usually vague. The 1580 pandemic was the first confidently identified as influenza. After that episode serious epidemics apparently occurred in Europe during the seventeenth century, but reliable, fairly detailed descriptions of pandemics cannot be found again until the eighteenth century.

Various workers have perceived the severity and spatial extent of influenza outbreaks from 1510 to 1892 differently. On the basis of overlapping agreement, six pandemics will be detailed: 1580, 1732–33, 1781–82, 1800–1803, 1847–48, and 1889–92. Records of the epidemics of 1830–33 are confusing, in part because medical observers were distracted by Europe's first great cholera epidemic, so those outbreaks will not be discussed here.

THE PANDEMIC OF 1580

During the summer of 1580, influenza was reported in Asia Minor and North Africa. Italian accounts suggest that it spread from Malta to Sicily in July 1580 and subsequently had diffused northward through the Italian peninsula by August.[15] The patterns shown in Figure 2.1 suggest a broad "clinical front" extending across the entire southern Mediterranean by July 1580, and this is in agreement with Hirsch's general statement that it spread from Africa and Asia simultaneously.[16] The western Mediterranean was then virtually a Spanish

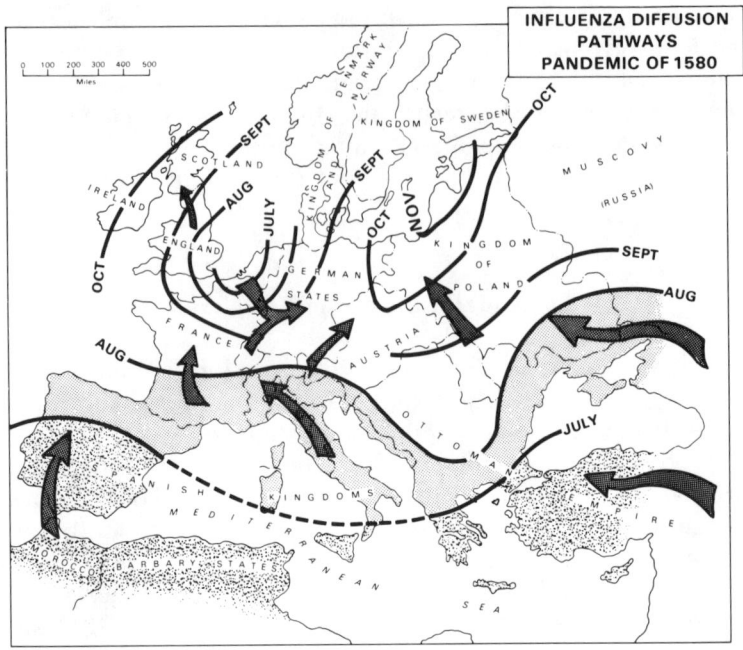

Figure 2.1. These postulated influenza diffusion pathways appear as a reflection of major lines of travel and communication in 1580, particularly within areas under control of the Spanish crown.

Hapsburg lake, with extensive commercial and political links that facilitated disease diffusion. Philip II, who ruled the Iberian Peninsula, southern Italy, and several North African ports, also controlled the Low Countries.[17] The early outbreak (July) in the Spanish Netherlands was probably caused by troops sent by Philip II to fight the rebellious Dutch. Indeed, the 1580 influenza can be called "Spanish flu" with much greater justification than that offered for the 1918–20 pandemic. The disease quickly jumped the English Channel from the Low Countries and diffused through the British Isles during August, September, and October. Influenza had broken out in Paris by September, and by October it had reached northern Poland. In the latter instance it appears to have spread from both western and southern Europe. Sweden and the eastern coast of the Baltic were not attacked until November.

Data for the late sixteenth and the entire seventeenth century are insufficient to draw any conclusions, but there clearly were serious epidemics in 1627–28, 1647, 1657–58, 1675, 1688, and 1693. The first two outbreaks may well have been facilitated by the devastation and military movements of the Thirty Years' War. Indeed, the entire period was marked by war and by expanding political and commercial contracts in Europe and between Europe and Africa, Asia, and the Americas. Influenza seems to have spread from Europe to North America and the Caribbean more than once.[18]

THE WESTWARD MARCH OF THE 1732–33 PANDEMIC

Two pandemics and several more localized outbreaks occurred in the eighteenth century. Italian accounts mention what appeared to be influenza during the winter of 1709, and outbreaks also occurred in France, Germany, and Denmark.[19] A somewhat more virulent form of what seems to have been influenza occurred in epidemic proportions in about the same areas in 1712. The 1730s were initiated with tandem epidemics, with the second (1732–33) being a true pandemic. While some sources contend that the epidemic of 1729–30 was the "first to originate in Russia,"[20] others note an interesting possible herald wave in Scandinavia during the early spring of 1729.[21] Mortality from that epidemic was particularly high in Italy and England in 1729–30. In addition, influenza was recorded for the first time in Iceland in 1730. It is difficult to tell whether the pandemic of 1732–33 was caused by a different virus or whether it was simply an extension of the earlier epidemic.

Indeed, accounts of the origins of the 1732–33 pandemic differ widely. Beveridge notes that influenza was probably present in New England in October 1732, and he contends that it reached Europe from North America, but Finkler indicates that both the 1729–30 and 1732–33 outbreaks spread to Europe from Russia. Hirsch's tabulations seem to confirm both notions, and the penetration patterns are consistent with this hypothesis of dual importations. However, while it is possible that the pandemic reached Europe from both east and west in the fall of 1732, another explanation seems more likely.

In 1732, in sharp contrast to the situation in 1580, Russia had extensive political and commercial contacts with western Europe, thanks in large measure to Peter the Great's modernizing policies. A 1721 treaty confirmed the transfer from Sweden to Russia of the eastern Baltic coast from Finland to Riga, giving Russia its first gateway to the West.[22] The extensive maritime trade in grain and naval stores that developed between England and Russia probably explains the rapid diffusion of influenza from the eastern Baltic to southern England. Although an introduction from North America cannot be ruled out, the 1732–33 pandemic might be labeled, at least from a western European viewpoint, "Russian flu."

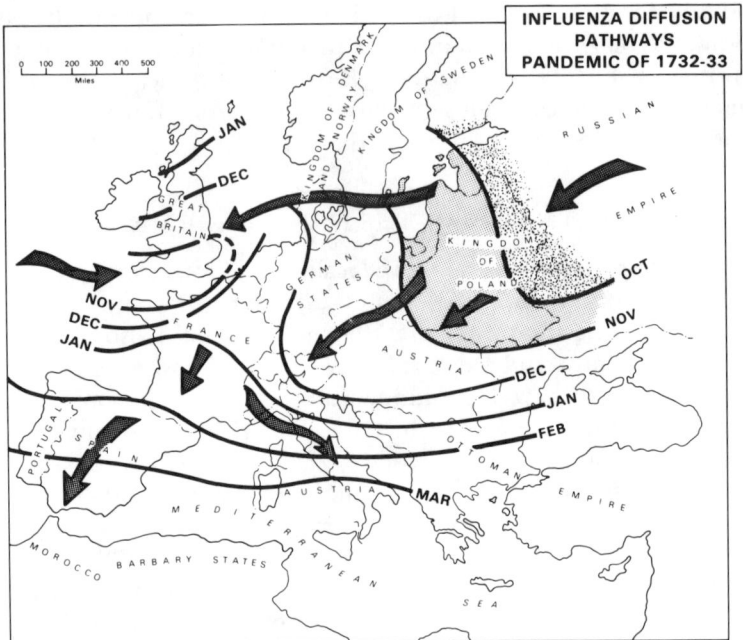

Figure 2.2. Even before the mid-eighteenth century, influenza pandemics seemed to originate in the Russian Empire as trade with western Europe increased.

As shown in Figure 2.2, the main wave moved into Europe from the east, covered Poland by November, spread through most of Austria and Germany by the end of the year, and had advanced southward to the Mediterranean by early spring. England was thoroughly infected by December, and influenza had spread northward to Scotland by January. Creighton's contention that Scotland was attacked before England is unsubstantiated.[23]

It is noteworthy that, although influenza reached pandemic proportions in 1732–33, it was not so severe clinically as the 1729–30 epidemic. This is consistent with the hypothesis that two distinct viral strains were involved and that the pandemic was not simply an extension of 1729–30 events.

There were no further influenza pandemics for fifty years. However, there were numerous outbreaks, some of which were extensive. The 1775–76 epidemic might, as Creighton argues, have originated in North America. In any event, it seems to have spread from west-central Europe to the Middle East, central Asia, and China—in other words, opposite the usual assumption of east-to-west diffusion.

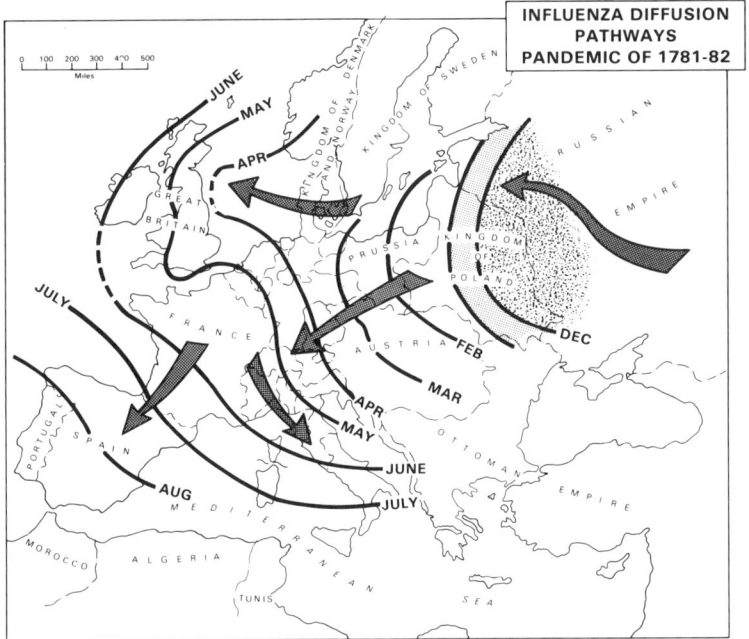

Figure 2.3. The pandemic of 1781–82 appears to have originated in the Orient.

THE PANDEMIC OF 1781–82

The pandemic of 1781–82 has some interesting features that invite comparisons with more recent related events:

1. There is some evidence of spring seeding, or "herald waves," in both Russia and North America in 1781.[24]
2. There was general diffusion of influenza into the Eastern Hemisphere later in 1781.
3. There were widespread outbreaks of what may have been a genetically shifted virus within China and British India in the autumn of 1781.
4. Following our current conventional beliefs, this possible altered agent resulted in a pandemic that started in China and spread westward in 1782.

Some sources indicate a fairly high young-adult attack rate. This is of course similar to what happened in 1918–20. However, case-mortality rates were much higher in 1918–20, so we can assume that the virus that was active in 1782 was considerably less virulent.[25] Still, the reconstructed diffusion patterns shown in Figure 2.3 cast a

familiar shadow. In spite of some suggestions that the disease originated in North America (a real possibility), the preponderance of
evidence supports the contention of central Asian origins. The "main
wave" of the epidemic in western Europe was during the spring of
1782; the pandemic had reached Moscow and St. Petersburg by
January.

Western Europeans were convinced that, as in 1580 and 1732,
influenza came from the east, but by now they looked beyond Russia
to China as the ultimate source. The disease seems to have spread
from Russia in two directions. A northern pathway can be identified,
with diffusion through Poland and Prussia during February and
March. Influenza spread rapidly through southern Scandinavia and,
probably again as a byproduct of the Baltic trade, had reached
Newcastle-upon-Tyne, England, by April 1782. The disease was
widespread within the British Isles by mid-summer. The other major
pathway appears to have been through south-central Europe, with
influenza reaching the western Mediterranean by late summer. Interestingly, there are only limited accounts of influenza in the Ottoman
Empire in 1782, although the disease was known to have occurred
there.

While contemporary observers often explained the spread of influenza in terms of prevailing miasmatic theories of disease causation, at
least one observer took a more modern contagionist view. Schönlein
noted that influenza took four days to reach Berlin from Konigsberg,
advancing as rapidly as a horse could travel.[26]

THE "NONPANDEMIC" OF 1803 AND THE PANDEMIC OF 1830–31

The nineteenth century began with an epidemic: During the autumn
of 1800 there was an outbreak of influenza in Russia, and by the
beginning of 1801 the epidemic seems to have settled in Germany
and parts of eastern Europe. During the same winter there were
outbreaks of influenza in China, but it may well have been caused by a
different viral strain. There were also reports of epidemic influenza
in Brazil at that time. By the winter of 1802–3 there were extensive
outbreaks in France,[27] and the disease seems radically to have diffused
outward from the French Republic in early spring. While some
authorities consider this episode a pandemic, it seems to have been
more localized, as with the patterns during previous winters (Fig. 2.4).

These events were almost certainly influenced by the Napoleonic
Wars. For example, in 1799 Russian troops were fighting in an anti-
French coalition as far west as Italy, Switzerland, and the Nether-
lands; the French counterattacked deep into Germany and Italy a

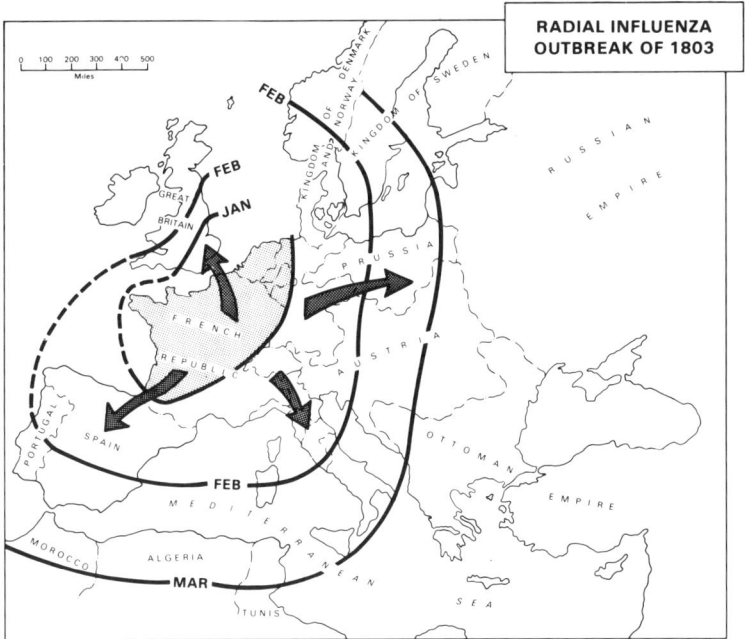

Figure 2.4. Some contemporary writers describe the influenza outbreak of 1803 as more serious than it seems to have been. Part of the confusion is because the pattern of radial diffusion shown here is only one in a series of such movements that took place over several winters.

year later. In March 1802 the Peace of Amiens signaled a fifteen-month lull in the wars.[28] French troops, pulled back from the far-flung battlefronts, retired to home barracks in the autumn of 1802. It is easy to imagine viral recombination occurring among the veterans, or among soldiers returning with infections acquired in eastern campaigns, with the new strain afflicting France in December with subsequent rapid radiation. Diffusion pathways through Great Britain can be reconstructed in some detail.[29] Earliest reports of outbreaks in January 1803 came from London, Newcastle, Dublin, and Liverpool. The disease appears to have spread radically from these nuclei. Some accounts indicate general movement from key urban places (mostly coastal) into the surrounding hinterlands.[30] This epidemic also appears to have attacked the elderly at a higher rate than the 1782 pandemic.

Influenza was again pandemic in 1830–33, but European data are deficient. However, the overall pattern closely fits current conventional beliefs regarding influenza pandemics:[31]

1. It probably started in China, since the earliest cases are recorded there for January 1830.
2. By the autumn of 1830, it had spread to the Philippines, Polynesia, and Siberia.
3. It diffused through Europe from east to west during the winter of 1830–31.
4. A second wave spread generally through Europe during the next winter.
5. It reached North America by the winter of 1831–32.
6. A second wave swept through Europe from east to west in the winter of 1832–33.

THE PANDEMIC OF 1847–48

The geographical origins of the pandemic of 1847–48 are unclear. There were minor epidemics in Europe for several winters prior to 1847, but the new outbreak had two significant differences: (1) mortality rates reported by contemporary observers were much higher than in previous winters; and (2) the influenza attack rate among the young was higher. Contemporary authors did not discuss a central Asian origin with an east-to-west sweep; instead, the pattern that emerges is somewhat similar to that of 1580.

The first reports came from the Ottoman Empire in August 1847. Two fronts then developed—one in western Europe and one in Russia. It is not clear whether these fronts represented separate epicenters, or whether ships brought influenza from the eastern Mediterranean to southern France in September. In any case, influenza had reached Denmark and southern England by October. This rapid overland spread was probably facilitated by the developing rail system of France and Germany. Influenza also seems to have spread north from Turkey into Russia, perhaps along river routes from the Black Sea, and then westward into Austria and the German states. The two fronts coalesced in central Europe by the end of 1847. In Great Britain early epicenters formed in London, Liverpool, and Edinburgh in October. This general multinuclear pattern can be associated with a virus that did not manifest a rapid rate of spread.

While all of the pandemics described in this chapter should be studied in detail using the primary sources, research on the 1847–48 outbreak seems especially significant. Preliminary data indicate a relatively slow advance, despite considerable improvements in transportation and an apparent spread from two epicenters.[32] This suggests a less virulent virus, with identification of separate epicenters possible because of its relatively slow movement. Diffusion of this type might also take place with more virulent strains, but it would be hard

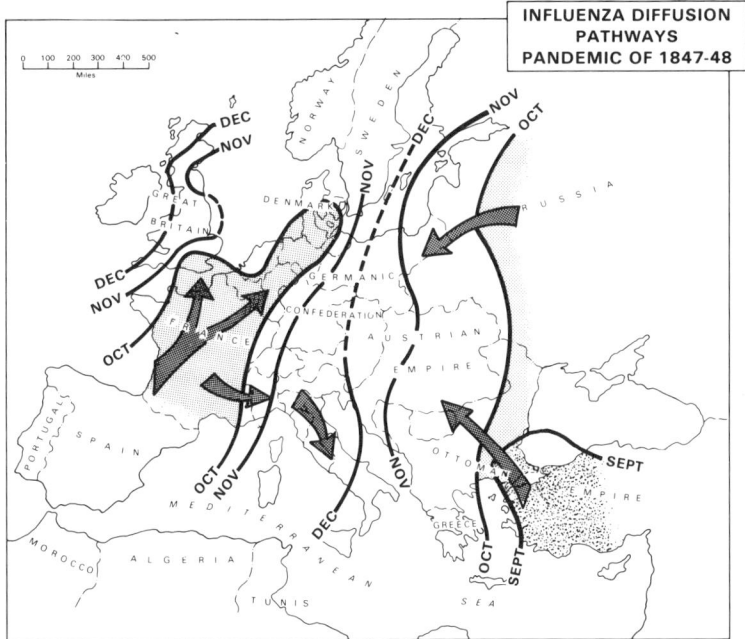

Figure 2.5. Accounts differ with regard to the origins of the pandemic of 1847–48; however, the postulated diffusion pathways within western Europe could have been related to the developing rail network.

to detect because the disease spread more rapidly. The behavior of the 1847–48 influenza seems to resemble the 1947–48 and 1980–81 epidemics in the United States (See Chapters 4 and 8), suggesting a possible historical relationship between the H1N1 viral strains.

THE PANDEMIC OF 1889–92

The pandemic of 1889–92, the last before the devastating 1918–19 outbreak, spread with great speed from its apparent origins in central Asia. In this and other features, the last of the Nineteenth-century pandemics bears considerable resemblance to the "Asian flu" of 1957–68. There was seeding or a herald-wave development in central Asia in the spring of 1889, followed by a characteristic summer lull and then extremely rapid diffusion through Russia into Germany and then into western Europe (see Fig. 2.6). This explosive spread was doubtlessly made possible by the extensive railroad network that connected Lisbon and London to Vienna and Moscow.[33] Indeed, for the first time in history, virtually all contemporary observers linked influenza diffusion to transportation networks.[34] The first wave was followed by at least two secondary waves.

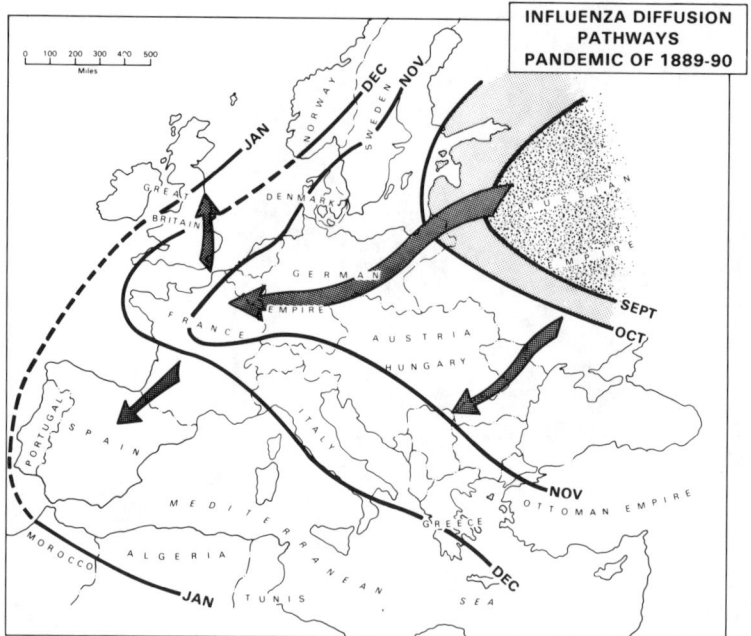

Figure 2.6. The railway network linkages in the late nineteenth century coupled with an influenza pandemic of probable Asiatic origins to produce the diffusion pathways shown here.

The initial wave had reached both North and South America by December 1889. Mortality in the United States was even higher the next winter, and a third, highly virulent outbreak was noted in January 1892. The pattern in Britain was similar: The initial wave of January-February 1890 was not especially virulent, but the second wave, April to September 1891, was more serious. The third and by far most devastating wave hit Britain during the winter of 1891–92.

Most medical observers agreed by the end of the 1892 pandemic that influenza was a contagious disease that advanced into new territory about as rapidly as human beings moved.[35] Older theories associating pandemics with the release of poisonous gases from the interior of the earth after earthquakes or volcanic eruptions or, more commonly, with noxious "miasmas" in the atmosphere held sway until well into the nineteenth century. Contagionism, supported by epidemiological studies on diphtheria, measles, cholera, and typhoid fever and by the development of the germ theory, was clearly ascendant by the 1860s. The last of the nineteenth-century pandemics was readily explainable by contagionist theory and was widely assumed to be caused by a living agent. Indeed, F. J. Pheiffer implicated a bacterium as a possible agent in 1890, and "Pheiffer's bacillus" remained a prime suspect for decades. The actual culprit was not discovered until the early 1930s.

One aspect of earlier beliefs remained intact: People continued to ascribe the origins of influenza to foreigners and often to non-Europeans.[36] This xenogenic (or perhaps xenophobic) theory was evident in 1889–92, when Europeans talked of the "Chinese distemper." Nationalism and political rivalries in Europe also led to such labels as "Nordische Ziep," "Spanische Ziep," "Calais Sweat," and "Scottish Rant." Flu, like syphillis, was usually blamed on foreigners.

Some General Forms of Influenza Diffusion

On the basis of our analysis of Europe's experience with influenza prior to 1900, the following typology of spatial diffusion patterns as models can be tested (see Fig. 2.7).

The Massive Frontal Movement Pattern. This pattern consists of rapid diffusion outward from one or several extensive source areas. The entire process of diffusion within an area the size of Europe may take only a few months, mortality rates can often be high, and a first wave is usually followed by one or two more. Subsequent diffusion waves do not necessarily follow the same pathways. Examples of this type include the pandemics of 1580, 1732–33, 1782, and the early 1830s.

The Multiple-Sequential Pattern. Also taking place within a single season initially, this pattern consists of multiple epicenter formation with outward radial expansion within a sequential temporal framework. Mortality rates are sometimes somewhat lower, and the youthful morbidity rate is often higher during such episodes. In general, diffusion rates are slower than massive frontal movements. The pandemic of 1847–48 seems to fit this pattern.

Seasonal Epicenter Relocation Pattern. Possibly not truly pandemic, this pattern consists of the relocation of diffusion epicenters from one season to the next. The European outbreak of 1803 appears to follow this postulated pattern.

The Herald-Explosion Pattern. This type of diffusion may actually consist of some combination of the other three patterns. In addition, there is evidence of spring seeding, or herald-wave development. This type of diffusion frequently begins with spring herald waves in "remote" locations that initially receive little attention because they

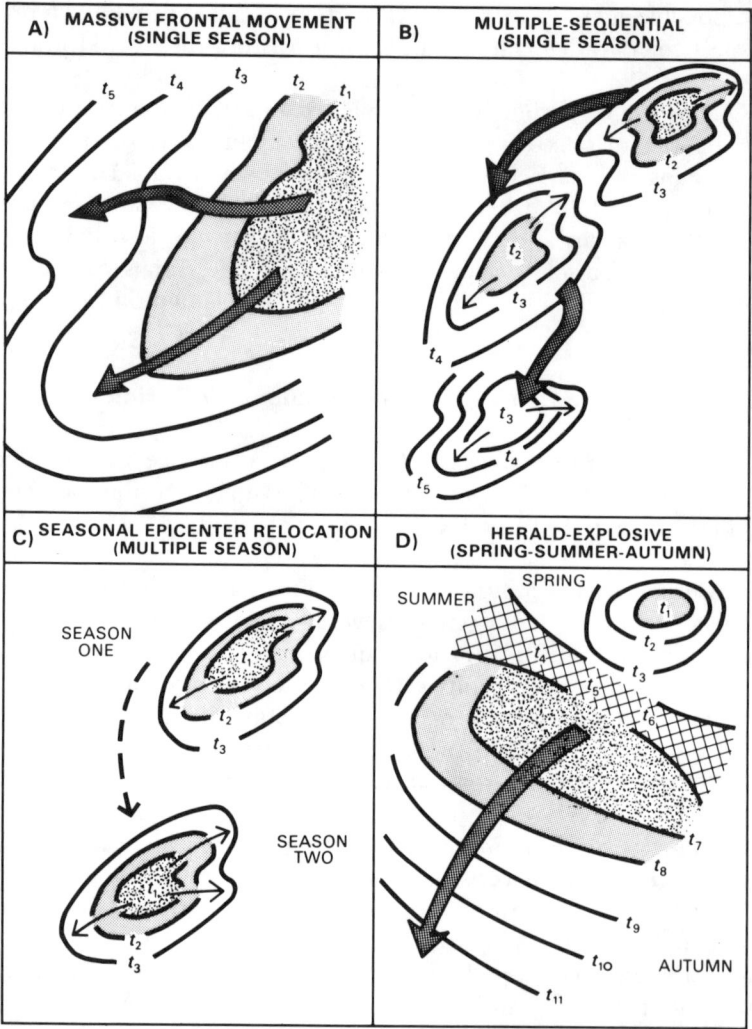

Figure 2.7. The evidence in this chapter strongly suggests this typology of influenza-diffusion possibilities.

appear to be mild. Influenza activity then seems to wane, but the lull is followed by explosive, massive diffusion across large distances within a few months. While the massive-frontal-movement pattern may be an extension of this type, the herald-explosion pattern is somewhat different because the explosive diffusion can take place in the late summer and early autumn rather than later in the year. Also, a second wave can develop later in the same autumn or during the following winter. The pandemic of 1889–92 seems to fit this pattern.

Two themes emerge from this survey. First, much of our conventional wisdom about the origin and diffusion of influenza pandemics can be traced to European notions of influenza as a xenogenic disease—one that always started somewhere else. This concept was well developed long before the 1918–20 pandemic or even before the discovery of the virus. The fact that the idea is old need not discredit it, but perhaps we look too readily to central Asia or China when we speculate on the origins of a particular epidemic. Second, and perhaps more important, this research suggests similarities between diffusion patterns of early epidemics and more recent ones for which we know the viral serotypes. These indications can only be tentative until more detailed research can be done, but a typology of diffusion patterns could lead to at least provisional serotype identification of earlier epidemics and pandemics. Such data would be very relevant to the debate over whether the influenza "A" virus has an almost endless variety of genetic permutations or whether a fairly small number of antigenic types are recycled.[37]

Notes

1. Alexander D. Langmuir, "Epidemiology of Asian Influenza," *American Review of Respiratory Diseases* 83 (1961), pp. 2–14.
2. K. David Patterson and Gerald F. Pyle, "The Diffusion of Influenza in Sub-Saharan Africa During the 1918–1919 Pandemic," *Social Science and Medicine* 17 (1983), pp. 1299–1307.
3. Alfred W. Crosby, Jr., *Epidemic and Peace, 1918* (Westport, Conn.: Greenwood Press, 1976).
4. W. I. B. Beveridge, *Influenza: The Last Great Plague: An Unfinished Story of Discovery* (New York: Prodist, 1977).
5. Gerald F. Pyle and K. David Patterson, "Influenza Diffusion in European History: Patterns and Paradigms," *Ecology of Disease* 2 (1984), pp. 173–84.
6. Robert E. Serfling, "Methods for Current Statistical Analysis of Excess Pneumonia-Influenza Deaths," *Public Health Reports* 78 (1963), pp. 494–506.
7. Edwin D. Kilbourne, "Influenza 1970: Unquestioned Answers, Unanswered Questions," *Archives of Environmental Health* 21 (1970), pp. 286–93.
8. Sir Charles Stuart-Harris, "Pandemic Influenza: An Unresolved Problem in Prevention," *Journal of Infectious Diseases* 122 (1970), pp. 108–15.
9. Selwyn D. Collins and Josephine Lehmann, "Trends and Epidemics of Influenza and Pneumonia, 1918–1951," *Public Health Reports* 66 (1951), pp. 1487–1516.
10. de St. Groth and S. Fazekas. "Evolution and Hierarchy of Influenza Viruses," *Archives of Environmental Health* 21 (1970), pp. 293–303.
11. Centers for Disease Control, "Influenza-Worldwide," *Morbidity and Mortality Weekly Report* 31 (1982), pp. 494–95.
12. R. G. Webster and W. G. Laver, "The Origin of Pandemic Influenza," *Bulletin, World Health Organization* 147 (1972), pp. 449–52.
13. August Hirsch, *Handbook of Geographical and Historical Pathology*, vol. 1 (London: New Sydenham Society, 1883), pp. 7–17.
14. Ditmar Finkler, "Influenza," *Twentieth-Century Practice: An International Encyclopedia of Modern Medical Science*, vol. 15 (New York: William Wood, 1898), pp. 3–249.
15. Ibid.
16. Hirsch, *Geographical and Historical Pathology*.

17. Geoffrey Parker, *The Dutch Revolt* (Ithaca, N.Y.: Cornell University Press, 1977), pp. 169–87.
18. John Duffy, *Epidemics in Colonial America* (Baton Rouge: Louisiana State University Press, 1953).
19. Finkler, "Influenza."
20. Ibid.
21. Hirsch, *Geographical and Historical Pathology.*
22. Warren Walsh, *Russia and The Soviet Union: A Modern History* (Ann Arbor: University of Michigan Press, 1958), p. 113.
23. Charles Creighton, *A History of Epidemics in Britain,* 2nd ed. (London: Frank Cass, 1965), pp. 359–85.
24. Beveridge, *Influenza.*
25. E. Symes Thompson, *Influenza or Epidemic Catarrhal Fever: An Historical Survey of Past Epidemics in Great Britain* (London: Percival and Co., 1890), pp. 142–43, 190–93.
26. Hirsch, *Geographical and Historical Pathology.*
27. Thompson, *Influenza or Epidemic Catarrhel Fever.*
28. Alfred Cobban, *A History of Modern France,* book 2 (New York: George Braziller, 1965), pp. 19–20, 44–45.
29. Theophilus Thompson, *Annals of Influenza or Epidemic Catarrhal Fever in Great Britain from 1510 to 1837* (London: The Sydenham Society, 1852).
30. Duffy, *Epidemics in Colonial America.*
31. Finkler, "Influenza."
32. Ibid.
33. John P. McKay, K. Hill Bennett, and John Buckler, *A History of Western Society,* 2nd ed. (Boston: Houghton Mifflin, 1983), p. 777.
33. Ibid.
34. F. M. Burnet and Ellen Clark, *Influenza: A Survey of the Last 50 Years in the Light of Modern Work on the Virus of Epidemic Influenza* (Melbourne: Macmillan, 1942), pp. 59–66.
35. Erwin H. Ackerknecht, "Anticongationism Between 1821 and 1867," *Bulletin of the History of Medicine* 26 (1948), pp. 562–93.
36. F. G. Crookshank, *Influenza: Essays by Several Authors* (London: William Heinemann, 1922).
37. Peter Palese and James F. Young, "Variation of Influenza A, B, and C Viruses," *Science* 115, pp. 1468–74.

3

Calamity and Discovery: The Early Twentieth Century

It was clear by the early twentieth century that influenza diffusion is contagious and that the disease can diffuse through urban hierarchies. In this chapter these ideas are intertwined in an examination of influenza before, during, and after the catastrophic pandemic of 1918–20. Discussions of the spread of influenza frequently refer to the calamitous epidemic that took place during World War I; however, in this chapter an alternative interpretation is offered of the spread of influenza within the United States during the autumn of 1918. Also, geographic aspects of the epidemic of 1928–29 are examined in detail for the first time, and comparisons are made with the previous epidemic. Since the latter epidemic was the last of any geographical magnitude prior to the discovery of the virus causing influenza in humans during the 1930s, the discussions of laboratory viruses in this chapter are based on the assumption that most workers were probably dealing with strains more closely related to the 1928–29 type of virus than that of 1918–20. Studies since the 1930s substantiate this assumption, and the pandemic of 1918–19 takes on an even more bizarre and anomalous nature when one examines demographic profiles of victims and finds that epidemics immediately prior to the "Great Pandemic" were more "normal" biologically because, in character, they resembled epidemics caused by more recently identified viruses.

Influenza Before and During the Progressive Era

The pandemic of 1889–92 is considered by many influenza epidemiologists to be the beginning of the "modern era," probably because it was the most severe epidemic since 1847–48 and beliefs about the contagious spread of disease were gaining credibility.[1] It is assumed that the disease spread through the more urbanized parts of the

United States as it did through Europe, but comprehensive data are sparse. Accounts from some cities and states, and demographic profiles of influenza victims as well as temporal aspects of separate waves in the United States, were similar to those of both Europe and Australia.[2] In his extensive treatise on influenza in the United States, Collins identified three successive waves of the disease in Massachusetts, beginning with an outbreak during the winter of 1889–90. The other two major waves, as shown in Figure 3.1, were during the spring of 1891 and the winter of 1891–92, the latter being the most severe of the three. In a description of the disease in Philadelphia based on clinical observations during the same period, Stengel also mentions three consecutive waves at about the same time.[4] The period immediately following the 1889–92 pandemic was characterized by temporal wintertime episodes similar to those described by Kilbourne[5] and discussed in Chapter 1. These episodes, termed "pseudo-influenza" by Stengel in 1918 and "trailer epidemics" by Burnet and Clark in 1942,[6] lasted until the turn of the century, when another, more important epidemic occurred in the United States. Still, little is recorded about the turn-of-the century epidemic, and it was apparently not part of a worldwide pandemic.

Sources do not agree on the temporal sequencing of influenza during the first fifteen years of the twentieth century, partially because epidemics did not occur during the same winters in various parts of the world, but also probably because the disease was not as serious a problem as it had been during the last decade of the nineteenth century. For example, Vaughn indicates general decreases until 1915,[7] but others suggest gradual increases in influenza mortality.[8] One common point of agreement is that during those times most of the victims were elderly.[9] The trends shown in Figure 3.1 for Massachusetts from 1899 to 1910 and in Figure 3.2 for a group of

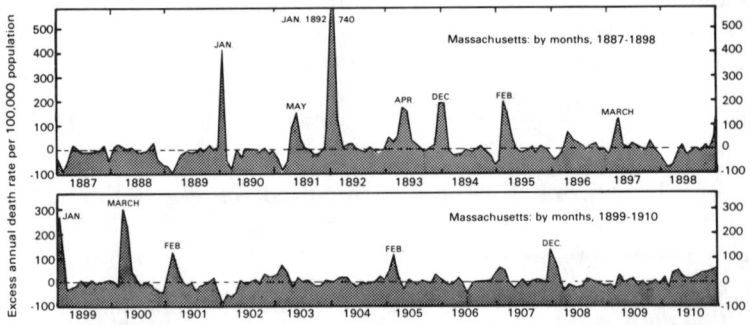

Figure 3.1. These temporal trends in Massachusetts indicate the severity of the influenza pandemic of 1889–92.

cities within the United States from 1910 to 1921 suggest occasional outbreaks prior to the Great Pandemic. This observation is substantiated by both Gill[10] and Jordan[11] in discussions of epidemics during the winters of 1900-1901, 1907–8, and 1915–16.

One remarkable coincidence of interest is that influenza activity increased in several parts of the world not long after the beginning of World War I. Apparent drifting of prevailing strains occurred as international travel increased. Most sources seem to agree that this condition resulted in gradual increases in influenza mortality throughout the world during the three winters prior to the devastating pandemic of 1918–20 (see Fig. 3.2).

We may never know for sure whether any of the changes in patterns of travel and other forms of human movement or displacement resulting from World War I led to the diffusion of any "precursor strain" to the Great Pandemic. "Purulent bronchitis" was common among British troops in France during the winter of 1916–17,[12] and it was apparently carried to India later in 1917.[13] Crosby also mentions the possibility of a "pneumonic plague" that may have been responsible for thousands of deaths in Manchuria and northern China in 1917, subsequently spread by Chinese migrant workers through the United States to France; however, United States public health records during this year do not indicate the diffusion of any such disease through the country. In addition, there are no indications of a central Asian or Chinese influenza-diffusion epicenter forming in 1917. Clinical records of that period indicate the presence of influenza on the basis of characteristic "U"-shaped influenza mortality curves. The influenza virus was not discovered until the 1930s, and many thought the cause of influenza to be the "Pfeiffer's bacillus" identified in influenza patients during the 1889–92 pandemic, and that organism

EXCESS ANNUAL DEATH RATE IN 35 U.S. CITIES 1910-1921

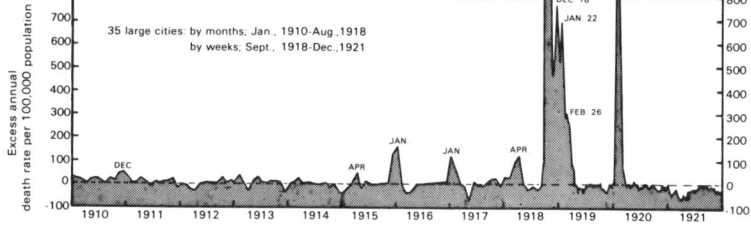

From Collins, Public Health Monograph No. 48

Figure 3.2. Using Collins's method, one can determine the impact of the pandemic of 1918–20 for a sample of thirty-five American cities. The disease was so severe during the autumn wave of 1918 that it was literally "off the top of the chart."

could be found later in victims of the 1918–19 pandemic as well as during the interpandemic period.[14] However, the nature of the Great Pandemic, both in terms of numbers of deaths and the ages of victims, was so drastically different from the outbreaks during the several preceding years that, once it struck, immediate priorities were more oriented toward disease control than searching for a casual agent.

The Origins of the Great Pandemic

Many retrospective analyses of the Great Pandemic suggest that it originated in the central areas of the North American continent early in the spring of 1918.[15,16] Agreement on this subject is far from complete, however, and there are accounts of influenza in China, Japan, and France in March 1918. The kind of influenza found in Kansas, Missouri, and other parts of the Midwest was somewhat different from the "ordinary form"[17] of the disease because mortality was characterized by a "W"-shaped age-morbidity curve. In other words, in addition to higher influenza death rates among the very young and elderly, there were also elevated rates within the 20-to-40-year-old group. It was not until the next wave of influenza during the autumn of 1918 that much attention was paid to the nature of the spring wave and how it differed from other epidemics in the proportions of victims who were young adults. During March and April of 1918, the disease spread from the Midwest into parts of the South and into many military camps in various parts of the United States. Probably, troops of the American Expeditionary Forces carried this form of influenza to Europe during the spring of 1918.[18] As the spring epidemic waned in the United States, an even more virulent form of influenza with the same "W"-shaped age-mortality curve surfaced in French port cities.[19] The disease quickly spread to the western front, which seemed to serve further as an epicenter for an incredibly lethal "second wave" of influenza that occurred in May 1918.

The Crack of Doom

The influenza pandemic of 1918–20 descended upon Europe in a ruinous fashion. As the disease spread from one army to another, it became known as "Spanish Influenza," perhaps because news from that neutral country was not censored during the war. But the disease had also taken a heavy toll of civilian lives in Spain by May of 1918, and it had also spread through much of the Mediterranean littoral.[20] It arrived in Scotland in May and was reported first in England in June.[21] As the initial, less virulent first wave of influenza waned within the United States, the altered and more merciless form continued to spread farther outward from its European epicenter, decimating many in its wake.[22] Mortality rates were high. In fact, it is on the basis of substantial increases in young adult deaths that pandemic pathways around the globe have been traced. Seasonal climatic variations seemed to have little effect on the progress of the disease, since there was little or no evidence of the transequatorial swings we can identify during influenza epidemics later in this century. The pandemic arrived in Australia later, probably because of the distance involved and quarantine procedures, but it was recorded in South Africa a few weeks after the first cases in West Africa.[23]

By August this more virulent form of the disease, normally considered as the "second wave" to avoid confusion with the milder spring outbreaks of 1918, had grimly cut its swath among populations of the Indian subcontinent,[24] Southeast Asia,[25] Japan, China, a large part of the Caribbean,[26] and parts of Central and South America. Thus, many of the lesser developed countries actually felt the impact of the second wave before the population of the United States. While the threat of the pandemic was clearly recognized by September, the second wave is thought to have first arrived in the United States in Boston in August 1918 (Fig. 3.3).

Researchers soon realized that this form of influenza was very different from kinds previously encountered. In addition to some of the classic symptoms of the disease—fever, headaches, nausea, muscle pains, and respiratory problems—many victims expectorated quantities of sputum and turned purple or blue. And sometimes this syndrome occurred within two days of onset of symptoms. Obviously not all who contracted the disease died, but many were severely ill. There were also repeated instances of a kind of lethargy that followed bouts of influenza.[27] Because of these circumstances and the high youthful mortality rate, many influenza researchers are of the opinion that the Great Pandemic consisted of more than one disease, perhaps caused by both an altered form of the agent responsible for the first wave and an additional pathogen.[28] Certainly a form of symbiosis could have occurred, but we may never know for sure. It is known that the pandemic led to the premature deaths of more than a half-million persons in the United States alone, and the international total, if truly known, would be in the millions.[29]

Given the annihilating propensity of the second wave, it is not difficult to reconstruct diffusion pathways within the United States during the autumn of 1918. One impediment to understanding fully

First Wave: 1918 Pandemic

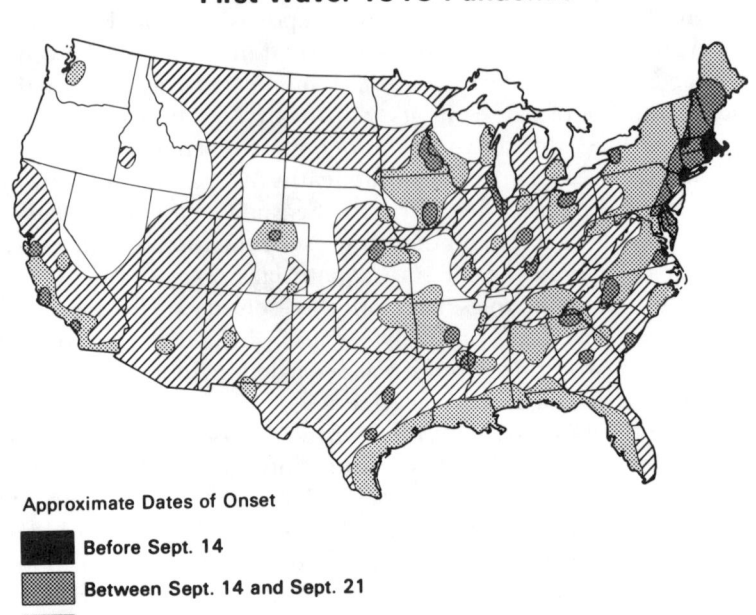

Approximate Dates of Onset

■ Before Sept. 14

▨ Between Sept. 14 and Sept. 21

□ Between Sept. 21 and Sept. 28

▨ Between Sept. 28 and Oct. 5

Figure 3.3. Sydenstricker's influenza activity map of late 1918. Although based on preliminary reports during the autumn of 1918, versions of this map have been reproduced in various public health accounts for almost seventy years.

the diffusion of the disease at that time was the explosive nature of outbreaks in different parts of the country (see Fig. 3.2). Since it was clearly so explosive, it took a public health network several weeks to formulate reporting procedures because it was not accustomed to reporting influenza mortality from specific cities on a regular basis. At the national level, one of the first comprehensive reports was released by William H. Davis, M.D., then chief satistician of the Bureau of the Census.[30] Davis used September 14, 1918, as a reasonable beginning date for weekly reporting of influenza mortality, with some allowance for cumulative pandemic deaths prior to that date. According to Davis and others who subsequently reported on the pandemic, the initial epicenter in the United States formed in Boston, with rapid diffusion to several New England cities and New York City. By late September several additional influenza epicenters had formed; these included the Chicago area, the Gulf Coast, and the Chesapeake Bay area (Fig. 3.3). Tables 3.1 and 3.2 show the diffusion of the disease during the early phases of the second wave in the form of recorded numbers of deaths reported within major cities, as well as estimated weekly mortality rates.

Some preliminary mapping of the progress of the pandemic was attempted by the Public Health Service in December 1918.[31] A map based on reports from military bases as well as several hundred urban places was produced, and it has been reproduced by several influenza researchers over the years, including Crosby[32] and Jordan.[33] Shown in Figure 3.3, the map conveys the impression of rapid, multiple epicenter formation, as is indicated by the following statements from the supporting text of the report:

> The outstanding fact, perhaps, is the extreme rapidity with which the epidemic spread after it attained the proportions of an epidemic in the first areas affected. The epidemic became nation-wide in four or five weeks after it appeared in an epidemic stage in the first localities affected. A fact of scarcely less importance is that the disease reached an epidemic state in a number of localities in the central, northern, southern, and western sections at about the same time as it did in the area along the northeastern coast. The possibility is suggested, therefore, that sources of infection existed in at least some of the larger population centers, well distributed through the country, some time before the disease appeared as a nation-wide epidemic. The apparent radial spread of the epidemic from certain centers would seem to strengthen this hypothesis. It may also be noted that there is evidence, the collection of which has not yet been completed, pointing to the existence of cases of the disease in various centers, probably widely distributed, weeks before they were definitely recognized as influenza. The possibility that these foci themselves had a common focus is by no means excluded, of course, but there is as yet no conclusive evidence that would warrant the statement that the starting point of the epidemic was Boston or any specific locality.[34]

That interpretation of the spread of the epidemic does not agree with either the pattern shown in Figure 3.3 or the data available at that time (Tables 3.1 and 3.2). The document also indicates that reports from about 175 cities were used to develop the map. Unfortunately, these data were apparently either not sent to the National Archives along with numerous other Public Health Service documents about the 1918 pandemic, or they were not retained in those files over the years.[35]

There is little doubt that the disease spread rapidly. In addition, most of the major "second wave" pathways can be identified by using reported influenza rates in developing a harmonic distribution for each of the cities in Table 3.2. (This method is discussed in mathematical detail in Chapter 8.) The mapping of most important harmonic phases for those key cities results in the pattern shown in Figure 3.4. Clearly a form of contagious radial diffusion took place during the

Table 3.1 Number of Cases of Influenza by City, September–January 1918
(weeks ending on dates shown)

	Estimated population 7/1/1918	September			October			
		14	21	28	5	12	19	26
Albany, N.Y.	112,565					45	110	186
Atlanta, Ga.	201,732					39	81	101
Baltimore, Md.	599,653				117	563	1,357	1,073
Birmingham, Ala.	197,670	2	2	5	16	61	110	133
Boston, Mass.	785,245	46	265	775	1,214	1,027	589	226
Buffalo, N.Y.	473,229				48	180	531	725
Cambridge, Mass.	111,432			105	140	115	63	21
Chicago, Ill.	2,596,681	16	24	91	417	1,047	2,105	2,367
Cincinnati, Ohio	418,022				18	67	192	281
Cleveland, Ohio	810,306				18	40	158	453
Columbus, Ohio	225,296					28	73	117
Dayton, Ohio	130,655					31	134	137
Denver, Colo.						59	129	147
Fall River, Mass.	128,392		9	20	97	201	192	97
Grand Rapids, Mich.	135,450						11	22
Indianapolis, Ind.	289,577					46	128	115
Jersey City, N.J.	318,770				66	231		425
Kansas City, Mo.	313,785				37	96	168	193
Los Angeles, Calif.	568,495					69	131	293
Louisville, Ky.	242,707					92	180	181
Lowell, Mass.	169,081			32	93	141	116	84
Memphis, Tenn.	154,759					80	182	166
Milwaukee, Wis.	453,841					69	113	175
Minneapolis, Minn.	383,442					48	99	150
Nashville, Tenn.	119,215					129	193	127
Newark, N.J.	428,684		6	8	53	189	396	431
New Haven, Conn.	154,865			15	36	77	152	183
New Orleans, La.	382,273				29	144	624	682
New York, N.Y.	5,215,879		106	191	733	2,121	4,227	5,222
Oakland, Calif.	214,200					18	42	138
Omaha, Nebr.	192,264					65	389	147
Philadelphia, Pa.	1,761,371				706	2,635	4,597	3,021
Pittsburgh, Pa.	593,335		17	34	69	114	389	576
Portland, Oreg.							41	94
Providence, R.I.	263,613				99	186	255	218
Richmond, Va.	160,719	4	3	4	41	131	197	128
Rochester, N.Y.	264,856					36	102	213
St. Louis, Mo.	779,951					86	186	233
St. Paul, Minn.	257,699					61	75	57
San Francisco, Calif.	478,530						130	552
Seattle, Wash.						75	108	160
Spokane, Wash.						4	19	
Syracuse, N.Y.	161,404			38	139	219	253	140
Toledo, Ohio	262,234					9	49	138
Washington, D.C.	401,681			34	173	488	622	389
Worcester, Mass.	173,650		17	101	199	230	160	89
Total		68	449	1,453	4,558	11,386	19,939	20,806

	November					December				January				Total
	2	9	16	23	30	7	14	21	28	4	11	18	25	
	155	52	20	4	14	7	11	11	13	12	12	8	11	671
														212
	397	147	41		40	58	68	74	57	48	75	83	150	4,358
	85	46	46	44	72	90		129	53	36	44	52	41	1,667
	137	76	47	54	54	63	83	132	201	244	227	158	153	5,771
	455	168	80	34	36	30	64	62	68	48		90	123	2,742
	19	5	9	9	7	6	14	17	26	39	22	20	16	653
	1,470	738	390	951	217	262	418	496	439	321	269	328	734	12,400
	248	163	97	105	94	149	2,208	163	83	51	18	18	26	1,981
	682	524	351	240	197	192	226	241	186	132	94	92	92	3,918
	94	50	36	43	64	98	83	59	21	15	14	10	20	825
	115	67	21		13	16	33	41	21	12	12	14	9	676
	108	101	77	108	132	184	201	163	86	65	47	35		1,652
	40	24	14	10	7	17	5	14	18	10	18	16	14	823
	18	13	29	22	18	30	51	38	23	18	8	8		309
	84	58	48	62	100	72	66	43	48	34	40	25		969
														722
	197	138	80	64	97	178	248	171	83	49	50	68	45	1,962
	382	309	300	196	167	125	134	141	117	99	151	178	177	2,969
	69	58	39	35	62	55	91	55	37	22	20	21	30	1,047
	30	8	8	11	2	10	10	8		13		20	26	612
	74		17	18			27	29		29			47	657
	125	95	70	49	88		182	166	105	65				1,302
	120	95	93	51	45	69	71	96	68	37	45	24		1,111
	51	53	15	16	23	26	28	29	22	20	17	21	21	794
	376	177	111	70	56	57	79	74	70	72	66	57		2,348
	168	82	48	20	24	32	30	52	36	40	38	27	26	1,086
	333	158	76	37	43	42	68	69	56	94	141	202	201	2,999
	4,462	2,277	1,053	657	424	446	477	534	678	753	870	998	1,193	27,362
	237	157	70	38	12	16	19	33	40	66	92	111		1,089
	94		68	68	34	92	155	141	57	29	25	17		3,081
	1,283	375	164	103	93	102	105	143	127	142	194	229	259	14,198
	638	798	532	385	297	200	202	144	127	99	103	111	145	4,972
	157	156	87	85	38	72	67	69	46	55	101	123	122	1,313
	135	65	36	33	23	34	39	45	64	47	59	62	61	1,461
	71	28	23	13	24	28	56	51		50	26	34	30	942
	209	104	52	40	37	49	65	87	73	59	26	17	21	1,190
	257	229	228	190	235	375	469	293	129	67	83	75	71	3,206
	102	109	135	88	69	68	65	64	41	39	25	14		1,012
	738	414	198	90	56	50	71	137	178	194	290	310	149	3,557
	109	85	69	34	47	77	117	103	78	55	70	57	57	1,301
	19	71	46	30	34	54	76	24	24	10		17		428
	68	28	23	7	7		9	11	8	8	13	4	14	989
	115	86	46	42	28	36	49	84	53	19	15	19	20	808
	181	55	42	37	42	41	86	120	154	139	109	107	73	2,892
	59		13	29	20	11	9	34	32	40	36	44	22	1,145
	14,818	8,442	5,038	3,492	3,192	3,619	4,635	4,650	3,846	3,483	3,565	3,924	4,199	125,562

Table 3.2 Influenza Mortality Rate, September–January 1918 (weeks ending on dates shown)

	Estimated population 7/1/1918	September			October			
		14	21	28	5	12	19	26
Albany, N.Y.	112,565					20.8	50.8	85.9
Atlanta, Ga.	201,732					7.7	20.9	26.0
Baltimore, Md.	599,653				10.1	48.8	117.7	93.0
Birmingham, Ala.	197,670	0.5	0.5	1.3	4.2	16.0	28.9	35.0
Boston, Mass.	785,245	3.0	17.5	51.3	80.4	68.0	39.0	15.0
Buffalo, N.Y.	473,229				5.3	19.8	53.3	79.7
Cambridge, Mass.	111,432			49.0	65.3	53.7	29.4	9.8
Chicago, Ill.	2,596,681	.3	.5	1.8	8.3	21.0	42.1	47.4
Cincinnati, Ohio	418,022				2.2	8.3	23.9	35.0
Cleveland, Ohio	810,305				1.2	2.6	10.1	29.1
Columbus, Ohio	225,296					6.5	16.8	27.0
Dayton, Ohio	130,655					12.3	53.3	54.5
Fall River, Mass.	128,392		3.6	8.1	39.3	81.4	77.8	39.3
Grand Rapids, Mich.	135,450						4.2	8.4
Indianapolis, Ind.	289,577					8.3	23.0	20.6
Jersey City, N.J.	318,770				10.8	37.7		69.3
Kansas City, Mo.	313,785				6.1	15.9	27.8	32.0
Los Angeles, Calif.	568,495					6.3	12.0	26.8
Louisville, Ky.	242,707					19.7	38.6	38.8
Lowell, Mass.	109,081			15.2	44.3	67.2	55.3	40.0
Memphis, Tenn.	154,759					26.9	61.1	55.8
Milwaukee, Wis.	453,481					7.9	13.0	20.1
Minneapolis, Minn.	383,442					6.5	13.4	20.3
Nashville, Tenn.	119,215					56.3	84.2	55.4
Newark, N.J.	428,684		.7	1.0	6.4	22.9	48.0	52.3
New Haven, Conn.	154,865			5.0	12.1	25.8	51.0	61.4
New Orleans, La.	382,273				3.9	19.6	84.9	92.8
New York, N.Y.	5,215,879		1.1	1.9	7.3	21.1	42.1	52.1
Oakland, Calif.	214,206					4.4	10.2	33.5
Omaha, Neb.	180,264					19.6	46.1	42.4
Philadelphia, Pa.	1,761,377				21.8	77.8	285.7	88.2
Pittsburgh, Pa.	593,305		1.5	3.0	6.0	10.0	34.1	50.5
Providence, R.I.	263,613				19.5	36.7	50.3	43.0
Richmond, Va.	160,719	13.	1.0	1.3	13.3	42.4	64.7	41.4
Rochester, N.Y.	264,856					7.1	20.0	41.8
St. Louis, Mo.	779,951					5.7	12.4	15.5
St. Paul, Minn.	257,699					12.3	15.1	11.5
San Francisco, Calif.	478,530						14.1	60.0
Syracuse, N.Y.	161,404			12.2	44.8	70.6	81.5	45.1
Toledo, Ohio	262,234					1.8	9.7	27.4
Washington, D.C.	401,681			4.4	22.4	63.2	80.5	50.4
Worcester, Mass.	173,650		5.1	30.2	59.6	68.9	47.9	26.6

Note: Figure in last column shows rate per 1,000 for the period reported, for each city.

November					December				January				
2	9	16	23	30	7	14	21	28	4	11	18	25	
71.6	24.0	9.2	1.8	6.5	3.2	5.1	5.1	6.0	5.5	5.5	3.7	5.1	19.4
34.4	12.7	4.4		3.5	5.0	5.9	6.4	4.9	4.2	6.5	7.2	13.0	23.6
22.4	12.1	12.1	11.6	18.9	23.7		33.9	13.9	9.5	11.6	13.7	10.8	14.8
9.1	5.9	3.1	3.6	3.6	4.2	5.5	8.7	13.3	16.2	15.0	10.5	10.1	19.1
50.0	18.5	8.8	3.7	4.0	3.3	7.0	6.8	7.5	5.3		9.9	13.5	18.8
8.9	2.3	4.2	4.2	3.3	2.8	6.5	7.9	12.1	18.2	10.3	9.3	7.5	16.9
29.4	14.8	7.8	5.0	4.3	5.2	8.4	9.9	8.8	6.4	5.4	6.6.	14.7	12.4
30.8	20.3	12.1	13.1	11.7	18.5	25.9	20.3	10.3	6.3	2.2	2.2	3.2	14.5
43.8	33.6	22.5	15.4	12.6	12.3	14.5	15.5	11.9	8.5	6.0	5.9	5.9	14.8
21.7	11.5	8.3	9.9	14.8	22.6	19.2	13.6	4.8	3.5	3.2	2.3	4.6	11.9
45.8	26.7	8.4		5.2	6.4	13.1	16.3	8.4	4.8	4.8	5.6	3.6	17.9
16.2	9.7	5.7	4.0	2.8	6.9	2.0	5.7	7.3	4.0	7.3	6.5	5.7	17.5
6.9	5.0	11.1	8.4	6.9	11.5	19.6	11.6	8.8	6.9	3.1	3.1		8.5
15.1	10.1	8.6	11.1	18.0	12.9	11.8	7.7	8.6	6.1	7.2	4.5		11.6
32.6	22.9	13.3	10.6	16.1	29.5	41.1	28.3	13.7	8.1	8.3	11.3	7.5	19.1
34.9	28.3	27.4	17.9	15.3	11.4	12.3	12.9	10.7	9.1	13.8	16.3	16.2	17.0
14.8	12.4	8.4	7.5	13.3	11.8	19.5	11.8	7.9	4.7	4.3	4.5	6.4	14.0
14.3	3.8	3.8	5.2	.9	4.8	4.8	3.8		6.2		9.5	12.4	18.2
28.9		5.7	6.0			9.1	9.7		6.7			15.8	
14.3	10.9	8.0	5.6	10.1		20.9	19.0	12.0	7.4				12.4
19.3	13.9	12.5	6.9	6.1	9.4	9.6	13.0	9.2	5.0	6.1	3.2		10.0
23.5	23.1	6.5	7.0	10.0	11.3	12.2	12.6	9.6	8.7	7.4	9.2	9.2	21.6
45.6	21.5	13.5	8.5	6.8	6.9	9.6	9.0	8.5	8.7	8.0	6.9		15.8
56.4	27.5	16.1	6.7	8.4	10.7	10.1	17.5	12.1	13.4	12.8	9.1	8.7	20.3
45.3	21.5	10.3	5.0	5.8	5.7	9.2	9.4	7.6	12.8	10.2	27.5	27.3	24.0
43.9	22.7	10.5	6.5	4.2	4.4	4.8	5.3	6.8	7.5	8.7	9.9	11.9	14.4
57.5	38.1	17.0	9.2	2.9	3.9	4.6	8.0	9.7	16.0	22.3	26.9		17.6
27.1		13.8	11.0	9.8	26.5	44.7	29.1	16.4	7.2	7.2	4.9		21.9
35.5	11.1	4.8	3.0	2.7	3.0	3.1	4.2	3.7	4.2	5.7	6.8	7.6	24.7
55.2	60.9	46.6	33.7	26.0	17.5	17.7	12.6	11.1	8.7	9.0	9.7	12.7	22.9
26.6	12.8	7.1	6.5	4.5	6.7	7.7	8.9	12.6	9.3	11.6	12.2	12.0	17.0
23.0	9.1	7.4	4.2	7.8	9.1	18.1	16.5		16.2	8.4	11.0	9.7	16.0
41.0	20.4	10.2	7.8	7.3	9.6	12.8	17.1	14.3	11.6	5.1	3.3	4.1	14.6
17.1	15.3	15.2	12.7	15.7	25.0	31.3	19.5	8.6	4.5	5.5	5.0	4.7	13.4
20.6	22.0	27.2	17.8	13.9	13.7	13.1	12.9	8.3	7.9	5.0	2.8		13.6
80.2	45.0	21.5	9.8	6.1	5.4	7.7	14.9	19.3	21.1	31.5	33.7	16.2	25.8
21.9	9.0	7.4	2.3	2.3		2.9	3.5	2.6	2.6	4.2	1.3	4.5	18.7
22.8	17.0	9.1	8.3	5.5	7.1	9.7	16.7	10.5	3.8	3.0	3.8	4.0	10.0
23.4	7.1	5.4	4.8	5.4	5.3	11.1	15.5	19.9	18.0	14.1	13.8	9.4	20.8
17.7		3.9	8.7	6.0	3.3	2.7	10.2	9.6	12.0	10.8	13.2	6.6	19.0

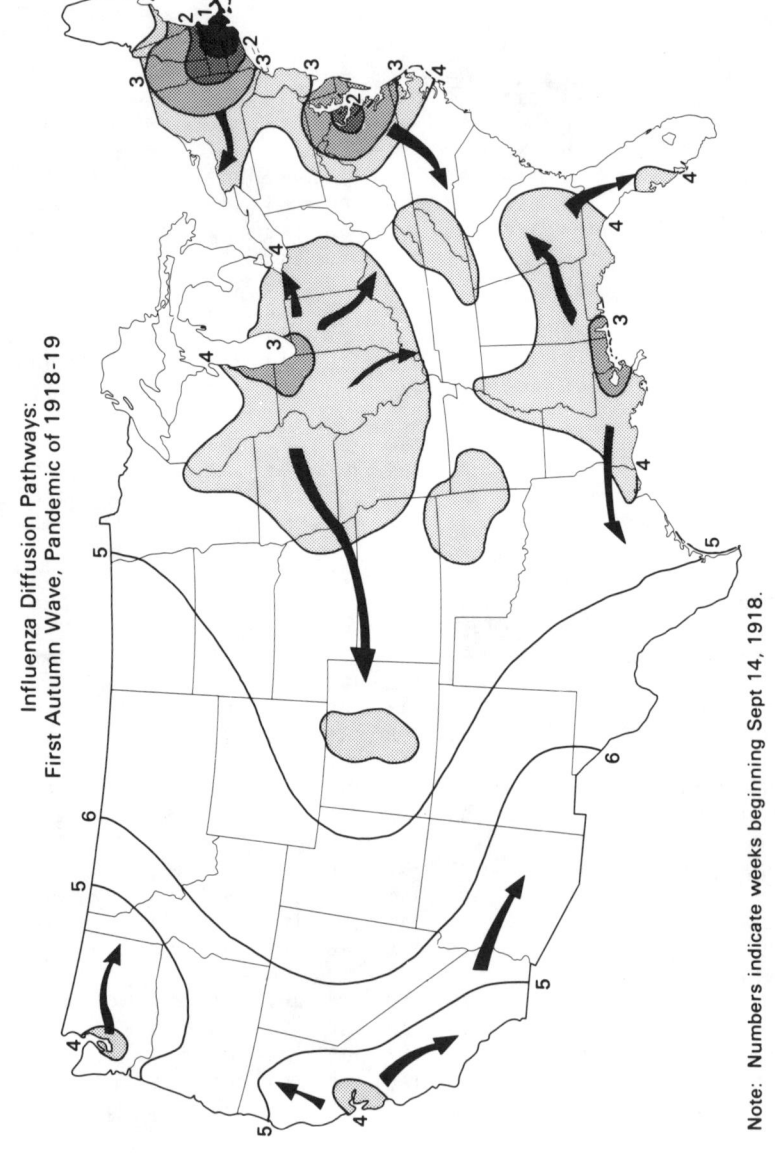

Influenza Diffusion Pathways:
First Autumn Wave, Pandemic of 1918-19

Note: Numbers indicate weeks beginning Sept 14, 1918.

Figure 3.4. The use of harmonic analysis (see Chapter 8) results in the pathways shown here. Both hierarchical and radial-contagious patterns emerge.

first wave, but hierarchial spread is also apparent as the disease seemed to skip from the very largest to next largest metropolitan centers. The patterns of diffusion within the southeastern parts of the United States probably were, in actuality, a little different from the pathways suggested using harmonic measures. As reported by Jordan in his 1927 analysis of the pandemic, the disease was widespread throughout the numerous army camps in that part of the country.[36] The third wave of the disease is more difficult to map. As indicated by the statistics in Tables 3.1 and 3.2, it was well established within the population by mid-winter, and influenza erupted from multiple epicenters during the third wave. Not all cities were affected in the same devastating manner, but the pandemic was generally so severe and different from past outbreaks that some common epidemiological aspects reported from various locales clearly stand out.

According to Pearl, a leading biostatistician and consultant to the Public Health Service during the early 1920s, four United States metropolitan centers that suffered particularly from the explosiveness of the second wave were Philadelphia, Baltimore, Washington, D.C., and San Francisco.[37] In fact, Philadelphia may have been one of the hardest-hit cities during the initial phases of the pandemic. The disease seems to have spread to the civilian population of that city from both the Philadelphia Navy Yard and Fort Dix, New Jersey.[38] While it was no doubt present in Philadelphia in September, influenza was not officially recognized as an epidemic until the first week of October. Within a month almost 11,000 deaths were attributed to the disease. The only American city to report more deaths during October 1918 was New York City (about 12,000 deaths), with several times the population of Philadelphia. While the actual number of deaths in San Francisco resulting from disease was lower than in some East Coast cities, that city had one of the highest morbidity rates on the West Coast. Crosby's account of influenza in San Francisco indicates that the disease was first known in September 1918.[39] This outbreak would be in keeping with the notion of diffusion of the disease to California via the Panama Canal. By mid-October more than 15,000 cases of the disease had been reported in San Francisco, but actual mortality from the second wave did not peak until November (Table 3.1). The third wave hit both Philadelphia and San Francisco in January 1919.[40]

Excellent statistics for Baltimore and a cross-sectional sample of other parts of Maryland during the pandemic are available from a series of civilian population surveys conducted and analyzed by Frost and Sydenstricker in 1919.[41] Using a total sample of 46,535, they found that 13,037, or 28 percent of those surveyed, probably had influenza during the pandemic. The case-fatality rate with 243 deaths was 1.9 per 100 for the entire sample and 2.0 per 100 for the city of Baltimore. The disease was first contracted in Baltimore during the first week of September, and it seems to have been part of the Chesapeake Bay area epicenter. With regard to age-cohort distributions, highest morbidity was found within the 5-to-9-, 10-to-14-, and 15-to-19-year-old groups. However, mortality rates were characterized by the "W"-shaped curve associated with the pandemic; that is, the hardest-hit cohorts were under 5, 20 to 40, and 70 to 74 years of age. The Maryland survey results also indicated that case fatality rates were higher for males in the broad 20-to-50-year-old cohort than for females of the same age.

In a detailed analysis of influenza mortality in Connecticut in 1918, Winslow and Rogers found patterns similar to those in Maryland.[42] Operating on the initial assumption that New London, with its naval facilities, was the epicenter for diffusion of influenza to the civilian population in that part of Connecticut beginning in the first week of September 1918, they discovered that mortality peaked within the state during mid-October. They further estimated that "excess" influenza deaths amounted to about 7,700 more than would be normally expected based upon the past several years' experience.[43] For example, the average October death rate in Connecticut from all causes for the 1913–18 period was 13.1 per 1,000. During October 1918, the influenza rate alone was 50.0. A number of surveys were also conducted by the Connecticut State Department of Health. Winslow and Rogers estimated on the basis of that information that morbidity rates varied from 200 to 400 per thousand persons, and fatality rates ranged from two to four per 100 cases. Another conclusion of general interest was that the incubation period seemed to be only about forty-eight hours. The age-specific morbidity and mortality statistics closely matched those uncovered during analysis of the Maryland data.

Similar statistics from Chicago also indicated the same kind of age-mortality curve, with the 20-to-40 age group being the most seriously affected.[44] According to representatives of the Chicago Board of Health, the disease diffused southward from the Great Lakes Naval Training Center in mid-September. During October, a peak month in that city, almost 6,000 people died from influenza. A strong indication of the relationship between morbidity and mortality in Chicago during the pandemic can be found in a 1919 study of three sample groups conducted by Jordan, Reed, and Fink.[45] The three groups they analyzed included the Chicago Telephone Company, which had health records for 7,500 employees, several hundred young men from the University of Chicago Student Army Training Corps, and another several hundred students and teachers from the elementary and high schools of the University of Chicago. The larger telephone-company sample indicated an overall morbidity rate of 19.2 percent and a case fatality rate of 1.5 per hundred. Given the nature of the pandemic and the fact that those employed by the telephone company were mostly adults, it was not surprising to find that the majority of cases were within the 16-to-30 age group for women and the 26-to-40-year-old male cohort. Statistics from the University of Chicago schools showed that morbidity rates were highest among the younger students. One of the two Student Army Training Corps groups of 234 men aged 20 to 22 years suffered two deaths, and nearly half of the cadets contracted influenza. The high attack rate was attributed to the fact that three students from that group were ill upon arrival at the university in mid-October. In general, major symptoms of the cadets who became ill during the epidemic included fever ranging from 100 to 104 degrees F., headache (66 percent), muscle pains (56 percent), sore throat (37 percent), cough (34 percent), and nosebleed (8 percent). Other accounts had included these symptoms along with some that were even more severe.

One of the most vivid of the many accounts of the disease written during those troubled times was supplied by D. G. Stine, M.D., of the University of Missouri.[46] When the university opened for the fall term at the beginning of September 1918, about half of the student body consisted of soldiers enrolled as a part of the Student Army Training Corps; they were mostly housed in barracks. The first influenza cases were admitted to the University Hospital on September 26, and from that date to December 6, 1,020 influenza cases were diagnosed. Fourteen of that total died. While a large proportion of the cases were not serious, some students were admitted in a state that Stine termed "toxic shock," characterized by subnormal temperature, low blood pressure, and mental apathy. Still others had developed inflamed external auditory canals, and many seemed to have a "characteristic sweetish smell" about them. More often than not, patients manifested weight loss over time, afternoon fever, night sweating, and sputum that was sometimes blood streaked. There were often other signs of internal bleeding as well, leading to increased chances of attack by secondary invaders. Stine expressed the view that the problem was not due to such agents alone:

> I saw one patient die within 18 hours of the onset of this disease and 12 hours after being put to bed. I have seen a number of others menaced with death during the first 48 hours of the disease. The statement that uncomplicated influenza cannot kill is, I believe, erroneous. It would be safe to say that death occurring within the first three days is due to influenza, and those occurring later are due to pneumonia or some other complication.[47]

In a further comparison of influenza during the fall of 1918 with the trailer epidemic of 1920, Stine observed that the disease of 1918 seemed to be "one of continuous infective process," while the latter seemed to be characterized first by a toxic phase followed by a pneumonic phase. The observations suggest that the agent(s) causing the Great Pandemic may have begun to go through some further genetic transformation as early as 1920.

Subsequent serologic studies of those who survived the Great Pandemic indicate that it was caused, as many suspected, by a virus. The sledgehammer effect of the event was the temporary flattening or indisposition and mandatory bedrest of approximately 25 percent of the United States population, but the agent(s) seemed to change and fortunately lose virulence over time. Epidemic waves continued until 1926,[48] and many now think that the responsible influenza virus ceased to circulate among humans at about that time and became what is now known as swine influenza.[49] Later, in 1976, the swine influenza virus was found in humans (Chapter 7), thus raising the apocalyptic specter of another Great Pandemic during the twentieth century. However, epidemics of influenza after the 1918–20 episodes appeared to be more "normal" than the Great Pandemic.

The Epidemic of 1928–29

Surprisingly little is written about the influenza epidemic that followed the Great Pandemic by a decade. By 1980s standards, the epidemic of 1928–29 would be considered severe because there were so many deaths from pneumonia as a complication of influenza as well as the disease itself. The Great Pandemic did encourage substantial laboratory research, and the Public Health Service continuously improved methods of influenza surveillance in the years following that disastrous event. Foremost among those who monitored nationwide influenza activity during the 1920s (and for that matter, the 1930s and 1940s) was Selwyn D. Collins. Initially in collaboration with some who had first established the United States surveillance system—Sydenstricker and Frost, for example, and later with others—Collins compiled extensive numerical comparisons that were used by an entire generation of influenza epidemiologists. The population of the nation had also become more urban than rural during the 1920s, thus making some of Collins's studies of groups of large cities during that period even more meaningful. One of the most comprehensive comparisons of the epidemic of 1928–29 with the Great Pandemic was published by Collins and some of his co-workers in 1930.[50]

The trailer effects of the Great Pandemic probably lasted until about 1926. During the spring of 1928 there was a surge of reporting of influenza-related mortality that may have been indicative of a herald wave, or "spring seeding" of a main wave, of epidemic influenza during the winter of 1928–29. These phenomena are shown in Figure 3.5, along with the trailer effects of the Great Pandemic and several follow-on wintertime outbreaks during the 1930s. These trends strongly suggest that some form of genetic shift had taken place in the late 1920s, and that an altered virus led to the diffusion of influenza through the country once again.

Before examining the probable spread of influenza in the United States in the late 1920s, one of Collins's major methods of measurement should be noted. Note that the oscillations depicted in Figure 3.5, and also in Figures 3.1 and 3.2, indicate rates above and sometimes below a zero baseline. Basically, Collins computed medians for key periods several years prior to major epidemics and then reported "excess" mortality rates over time.[51] This comparative measurement system proved to be quite useful for several decades. When medical improvements during the 1940s resulted in substantial declines in pneumonia deaths, P&I mortality statistics followed a similar trend. The Collins method thus failed to "predict" the 1957 epidemic, and more sophisticated methods were then developed for influenza surveillance (see Chapter 5).

The Collins method works well for comparisons of early twentieth-century influenza epidemics. For example, the statistics in Table 3.3 help in understanding spatio-temporal similarities and differences in excess P&I mortality rates per 100,000 population during an era when more deaths resulted from these conditions than at present. The mortality rates reported for the Great Pandemic were so high that they seem to overshadow those from the epidemic of 1928–29. However, the latter episode was more severe than the several winters before the pandemic of 1918–20. The statistics in Table 3.3 have also been computed so that spring herald waves can be compared. In

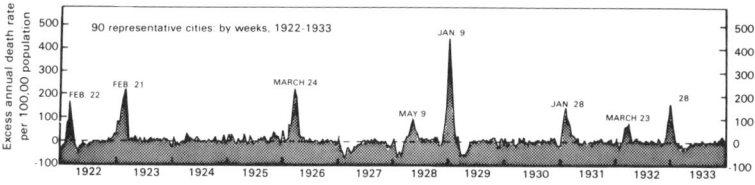

Figure 3.5. As shown in this graph, the most severe influenza epidemic to take place after the "trailer" effects of the 1918–20 pandemic occurred during the winter of 1928–29.

Table 3.3   Total Excess Mortality from Influenza and Pneumonia per 100,000 population in Each of Fifty Large U.S. Cities (arranged geographically), 1910–29

	1915	1916	1917	Spring 1918	Winter 1918–19	1920	1922	1923	1925	1926	Spring 1928	Winter 1928–29
Boston	6.0	36.1	25.3	34.1	686.5	98.8	24.3	53.0	15.0	24.7	20.2	53.1
Providence	20.7	33.5	33.7	29.0	618.0	103.2	27.8	29.5	6.9	22.9	9.8	34.7
New Haven	7.8	38.7	25.6	22.5	583.7	122.7	39.1	30.3	7.	19.3	31.6	22.3
Albany	27.1	32.5	11.5	8.0	589.0	57.2	32.4	58.7	6.0	41.8	19.2	65.8
Buffalo	14.9	17.1	26.3	21.7	531.1	85.8	13.9	29.8	8.8	34.0	22.0	63.8
New York	8.1	20.0	17.2	23.3	462.6	97.1	23.7	23.1	12.2	36.2	33.5	42.3
Rochester	8.4	0	21.4	23.8	394.3	44.4	20.5	26.7	4.3	44.9	4.2	21.4
Syracuse	8.7	13.3	10.3	37.7	454.1	136.9	0	30.2	12.2	21.8	24.9	59.0
Jersey City	19.5	34.2	24.0	41.4	664.0	103.3	16.0	22.4	5.4	39.3	33.6	41.4
Newark	5.9	24.2	28.7	45.4	551.4	103.8	20.3	28.8	8.5	30.9	22.2	44.6
Paterson	0	48.8	24.2	12.4	612.4	70.5	36.6	36.4	10.8	32.3	15.3	38.3
Philadelphia	11.7	52.7	60.0	77.8	708.5	88.5	5.5	41.7	6.9	34.9	11.1	34.3
Pittsburgh	8.7	86.9	88.8	192.0	1,008.7	147.2	24.4	90.0	2.2	9.5	14.4	127.62
Scranton	12.9	23.8	28.6	64.2	753.5	122.2	28.2	26.4	50.4	28.2	09.3	14.6
Baltimore	11.3	39.4	24.9	39.2	632.9	73.5	1.6	30.6	13.9	30.6	14.1	45.9
Washington, D.C.	30.5	21.1	15.1	49.9	572.3	106.7	0	83.2	0	22.7	3.4	27.5
Richmond	12.1	34.9	15.9	9.7	551.3	74.0	4.9	14.5	0	60.9	4.4	44.0
Atlanta	5.6	0	0	71.7	358.7	128.0	14.6	42.4	38.2	10.5	6.8	86.6
Cincinnati	6.4	27.5	18.0	33.6	534.8	70.2	26.0	47.3	20.3	38.4	23.7	70.5
Cleveland	13.3	61.8	68.8	44.8	568.2	87.3	7.9	23.9	3.6	36.1	9.5	53.6
Columbus	9.9	44.2	34.4	16.0	368.1	139.7	15.1	85.9	40.7	7.9	5.5	79.6
Dayton	10.7	15.2	10.0	14.4	420.3	86.5	5.4	49.2	15.4	26.5	13.7	38.4

City											
Toledo	7.5	40.2	45.2	20.1	350.6	74.1	13.2	28.0	6.3	17.3	20.0	65.8
Indianapolis	16.0	23.5	12.7	38.4	392.8	118.2	29.6	41.2	23.7	17.8	29.0	70.9
Chicago	0	22.0	12.0	6.9	380.5	112.8	0	23.2	0	16.3	23.5	30.5
Detroit	0	20.4	42.3	24.0	338.0	108.3	17.6	51.7	0	57.0	15.0	45.5
Grand Rapids	22.4	18.0	9.9	22.5	198.5	74.7	6.4	57.4	9.3	18.5	10.4	51.5
Milwaukee	13.6	57.0	63.4	33.1	368.4	111.1	0	31.4	22.3	21.6	26.7	46.0
Louisville	20.7	37.1	32.7	87.2	611.4	32.0	16.3	34.4	3.7	45.8	28.4	52.0
Memphis	0	29.2	29.1	40.0	565.3	97.9	11.2	76.8	21.9	9.4	9.4	95.0
Nashville	0	10.2	0	124.9	688.0	121.8	10.8	65.8	3.3	93.1	43.1	81.7
Birmingham	0	8.2	100.2	195.0	643.4	135.3	0	6.2	71.2	84.3	46.9	137.4
Minneapolis	0	28.0	16.6	31.9	310.0	103.3	7.9	10.6	15.0	18.8	16.0	38.0
St. Paul	8.7	22.4	14.1	25.3	385.3	94.5	12.4	28.8	13.2	6.8	61.8	69.9
Omaha	7.4	71.5	71.8	29.8	550.8	102.7	16.3	40.3	12.6	14.6	6.7	50.7
Kansas City, Mo.	13.5	37.9	65.2	76.1	652.3	205.3	29.0	38.3	21.0	8.3	5.7	41.6
St. Louis	0	39.0	59.5	41.0	384.8	113.9	20.0	20.6	8.4	20.9	17.6	30.4
New Orleans	27.5	20.3	7.9	21.9	709.3	62.6	7.8	9.1	8.7	44.1	36.0	85.3
Denver	12.2	42.7	13.8	50.2	629.7	138.4	20.3	18.5	25.3	6.7	12.0	86.5
Los Angeles	0	7.1	0	0	500.7	29.6	30.9	7.3	4.8	4.5	17.9	79.4
Oakland	0	3.9	7.6	25.0	507.3	92.6	18.0	11.0	0	6.8	16.2	29.2
San Francisco	0	0	5.4	22.7	635.6	93.6	35.4	14.9	3.8	8.9	3.9	6.8
Portland, Oreg.	0	6.9	9.0	37.0	505.9	67.5	38.3	22.9	6.5	4.3	0	33.7
Seattle	6.3	0	4.2	27.2	419.9	89.7	17.6	0	7.4	9.0	0	42.7
Spokane	0	9.5	18.2	12.4	490.4	126.6	39.3	0	5.5	12.0	20.4	89.6

Note: "Excess mortality" signifies excess over the median monthly rate for the period 1910–16 for epidemics prior to July 1, 1919, and excess over the median monthly rate for the period 1921–27 for epidemics after July 1, 1919. The period considered as epidemic varied in the different cities, all positive deviations being included for months when the rate was above the median.

almost all of the cities listed, this phenomenon seems to have taken place during the Great Pandemic as well as during the epidemic of 1928–29, but in many cities the excess rate in the spring of 1918 was actually higher by about 20 percent than the similar rate for the wintertime epidemic of 1928–29.

Our legacy from the "Collins era" includes even more detailed monthly reporting of influenza deaths by major cities.[52] Such information can be used to test some of the paradigms that had developed by then. There is no absolute scientific proof that the first wave of the Great Pandemic was the "milder" form of influenza that erupted during the spring of 1918. (Another examination of Table 3.3 leads once again to the conclusion it was "seeded".) The popular "Spanish Influenza" label seemed to prevail; the disease had come from someplace else.

What about the epidemic of 1928–29? Figures 3.6 to 3.11 test the xenogenic paradigm for that event. The proportional circles of these maps indicate the numbers of influenza deaths reported during the various months. Cities are initially introduced into the diffusion system and placed on the monthly maps when there are clear indications of upward trends; that is, definite and sustained increases in influenza reporting. Thus, the sequence of monthly maps in Figures 3.6 and 3.7 initially depicts the increasing temporal magnitude of the problem during the spring of 1928. In addition, the shaded circles indicate numerical peaks; this peaking frequently corresponds to the fiftieth percentile of a given temporal distribution. (In this instance, only the springtime distribution is considered.) The sequence of maps in Figures 3.6 and 3.7 gives the general impression that if an altered influenza virus were introduced into the United States from some extraneous source, it probably happened during the late autumn of 1927 because, by January 1928, most of the major cities of the Northeastern Seaboard and several farther inland had indicated an upward trend in reporting. The disease seems to have spread quickly into the Midwest and then had diffused westward by April 1928. It is important to note that Collins did not indicate a spring 1928 nationwide peak until May 1928, but according to this analysis the possible seeding phase had by then already begun to wane.

Influenza mortality reporting continued to decline in many places during the summer of 1928, but as early as July some cities in the Ohio Valley, New York, the Midwest (Omaha), and California indicated widespread summertime increases (Fig. 3.8 and 3.9). Reporting of influenza mortality continued to show a slow but steady increase in scattered locations during August and September of 1928, and by September most major cities within the country had indicated general increases in the disease ordinarily expected in autumn. The epidemic did not actually reach explosive proportions until December and January. As shown in Figure 3.10, epicenters had formed in the Pacific Northwest, California, the Southeast, and several midwestern locations by November 1928. By December, most of the larger reporting cities west of the 100th Meridian had reached epidemic peaks along with many of the midwestern cities that had previously indicated early epidemic beginnings. Most of the Northeastern Seaboard locations that had reported extensive numbers of influenza cases during the spring lagged behind cities farther to the west with regard to peak reporting. The Southeast seems to have been a special case during both waves of this epidemic. There were unusually high numbers of influenza deaths in Memphis, Nashville, Birmingham, and Atlanta during April 1928, and these four cities, after somewhat of a lag during the autumn, again reported high numbers of influenza deaths, especially during January 1928. For some reason, Birmingham alone reported almost 1,800 influenza deaths that month.

An examination of the autumn-winter patterns alone gives the impression of a general west-midwest to east-southeast diffusion pathway system during the 1928–29 epidemic, but when the 1928 springtime patterns are reexamined in light of the autumn second wave, just the opposite seems to have been the case. In other words, the virus may have entered the country from the east and initially spread to the west. It then gradually reversed its course and perhaps as a result of the balance between immunes and susceptibles reached epidemic proportions later in those locations it had visited earlier. The possibility exists that the virus discovered in the early 1930s was one that entered the country in late 1927 or early 1928, caused the rather bad epidemic of 1928–29, and then formed several trailer outbreaks during the early 1930s (Fig. 3.5).

Some of the strongest evidence supporting the argument that the 1928–29 virus was different from that of the Great Pandemic is data in the form of the ages of those who died during the epidemics.[53] In addition to extreme differences in the actual numbers of deaths from the first to the second epidemic, the "W"-shaped age-mortality curve of the pandemic of 1918–20 did not show up during the epidemic of 1928–29. A comparison of the two epidemics is shown in Figure 3.12. During the 1928–29 epidemic, the highest mortality rates were among the elderly, while during the earlier episode, the 20-to-40-year-old cohort was especially victimized. The virus that was discovered in humans during the early 1930s was probably more closely related to the 1928–29 type than the earlier agent, and the latter strain seems to have been of geographically extraneous origin.

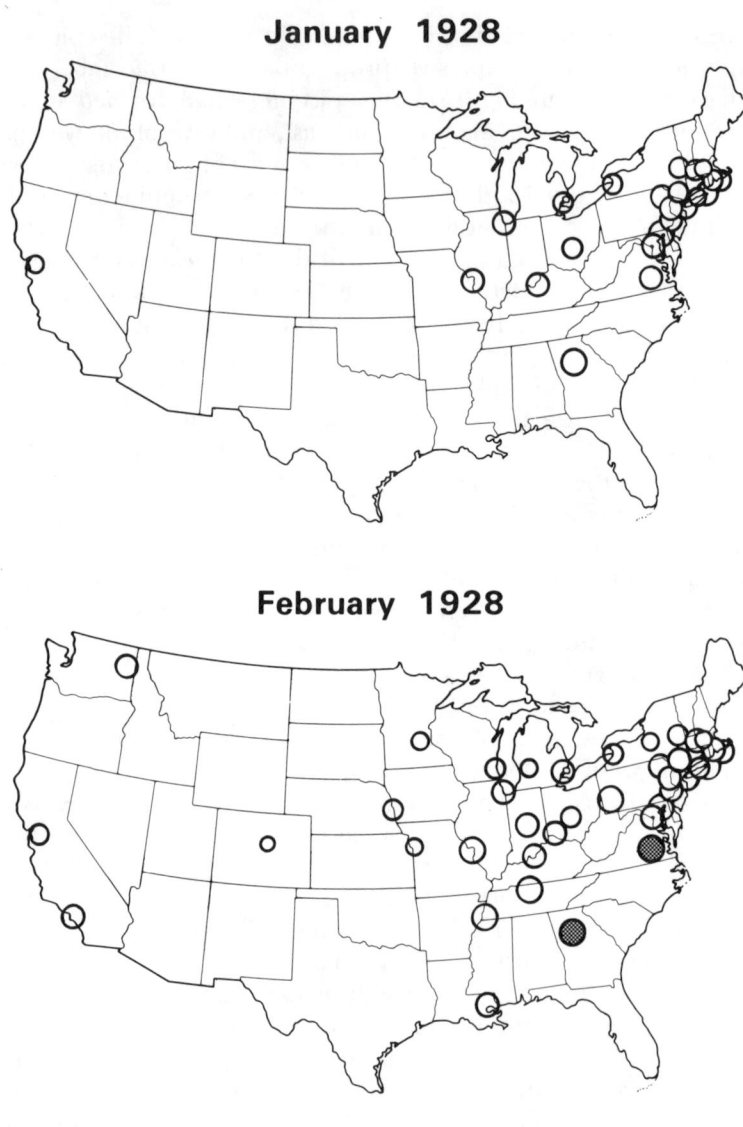

Figure 3.6. The influenza outbreak in January and February 1928 seems to have had more than one epicenter. The shaded circles indicate a springtime peak.

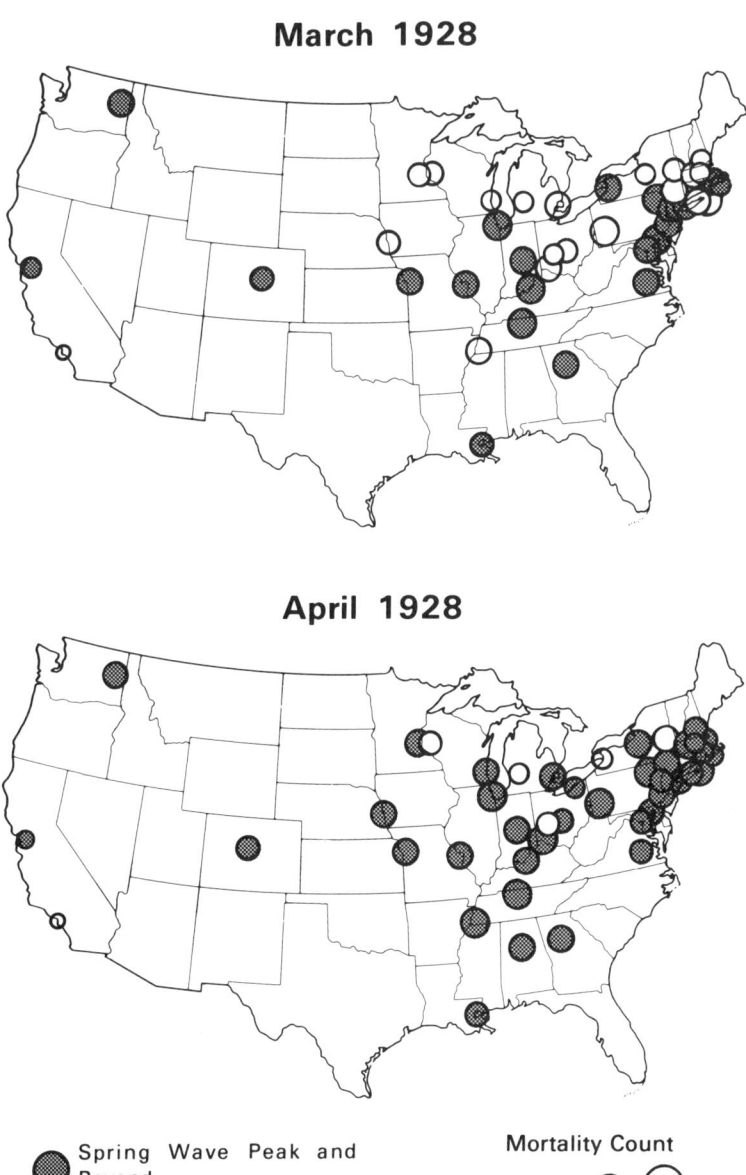

Figure 3.7. These maps show how influenza spread from epicenters during the spring of 1928.

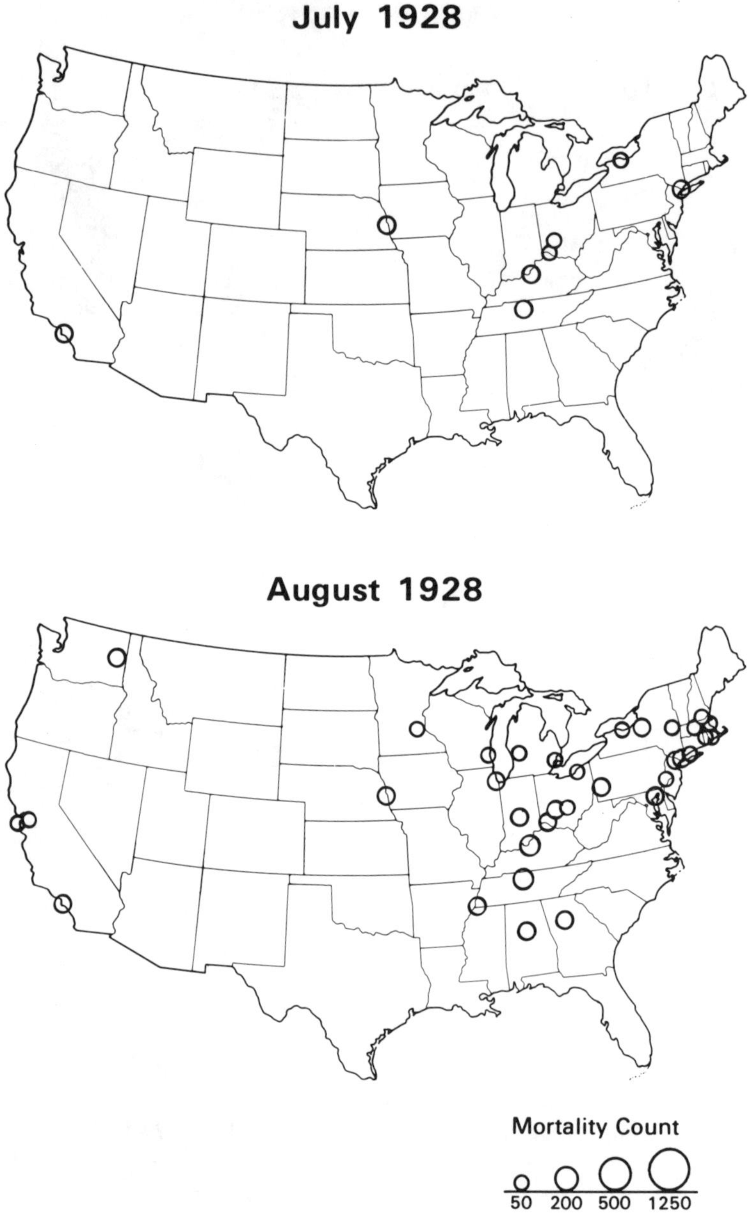

July 1928

August 1928

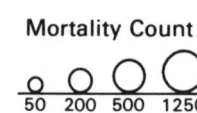

Mortality Count

50   200   500   1250

Figure 3.8. During the summer of 1928, influenza began to spread from the interior of the country.

September 1928

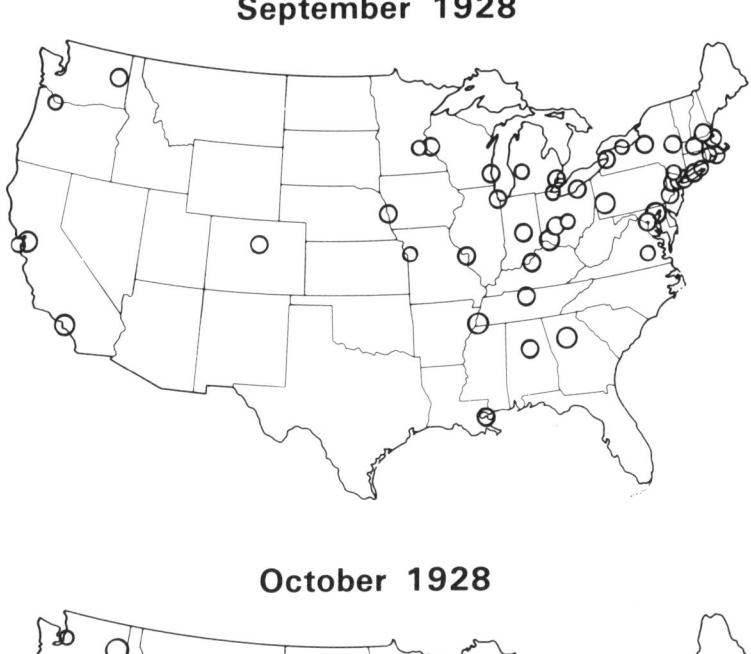

October 1928

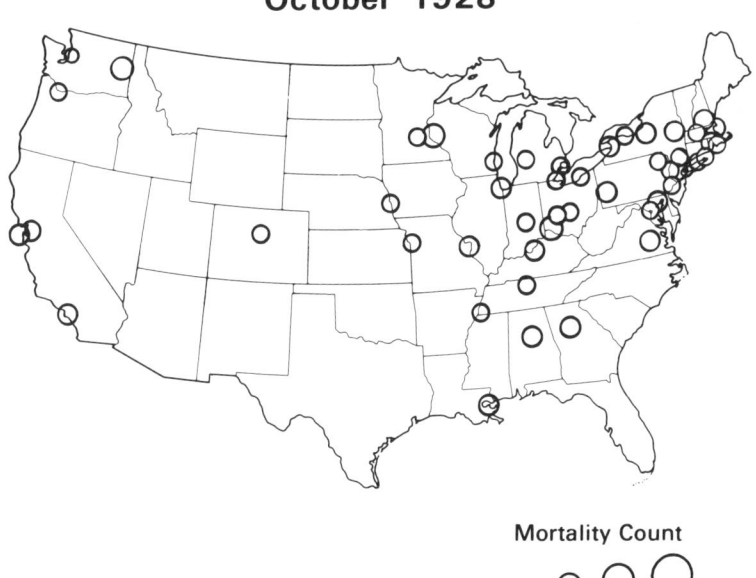

Mortality Count

50 200 500 1250

Figure 3.9. Influenza continued to spread from mid-summer epicenters during the early autumn 1928.

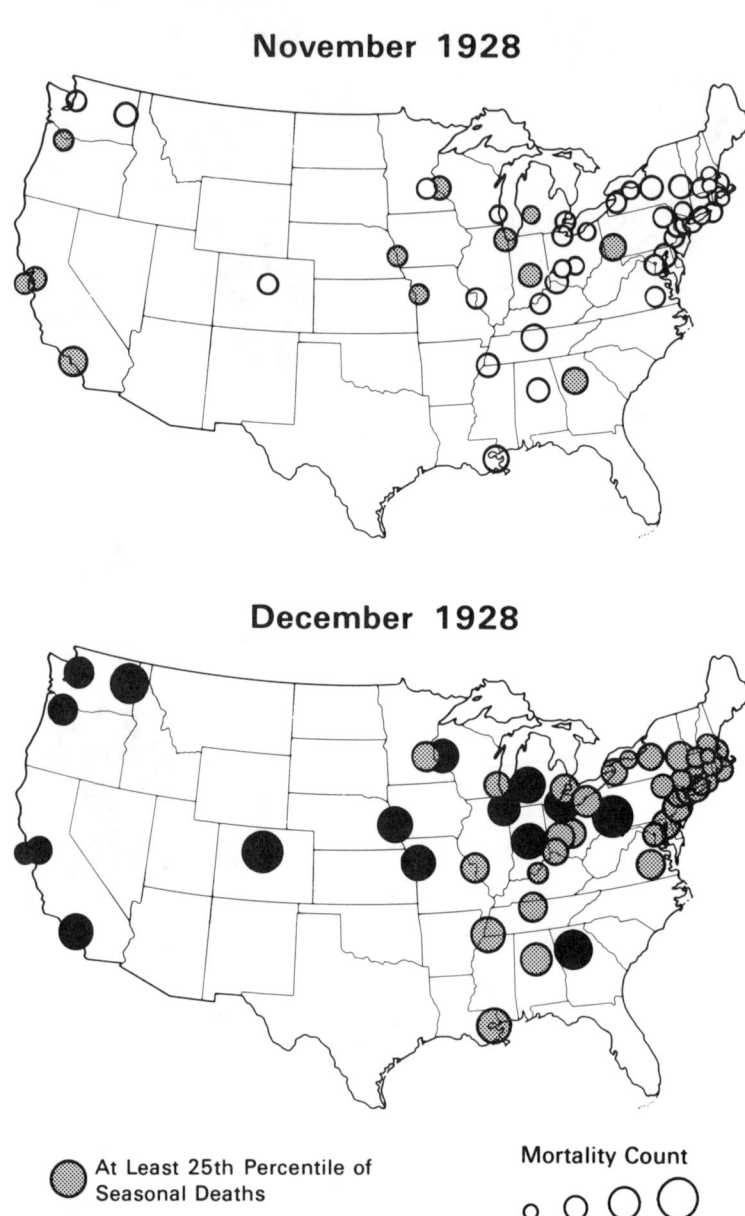

November 1928

December 1928

At Least 25th Percentile of Seasonal Deaths

Exceeding 50th Percentile

Mortality Count

50   200   500   1250

Figure 3.10. By the late fall and early winter of 1928–29, influenza deaths began to peak in many interior and west coast cities.

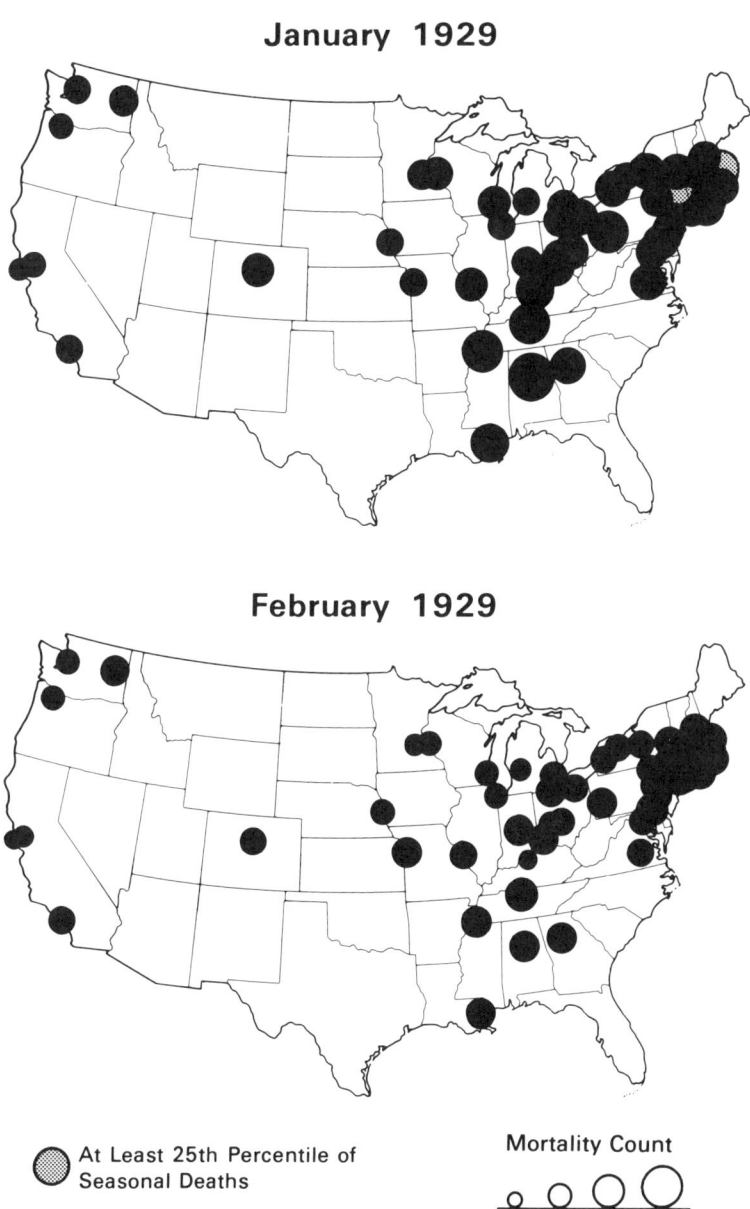

Figure 3.11. Influenza mortality had peaked and begun to decline in most parts of the United States by the late winter of 1928–29.

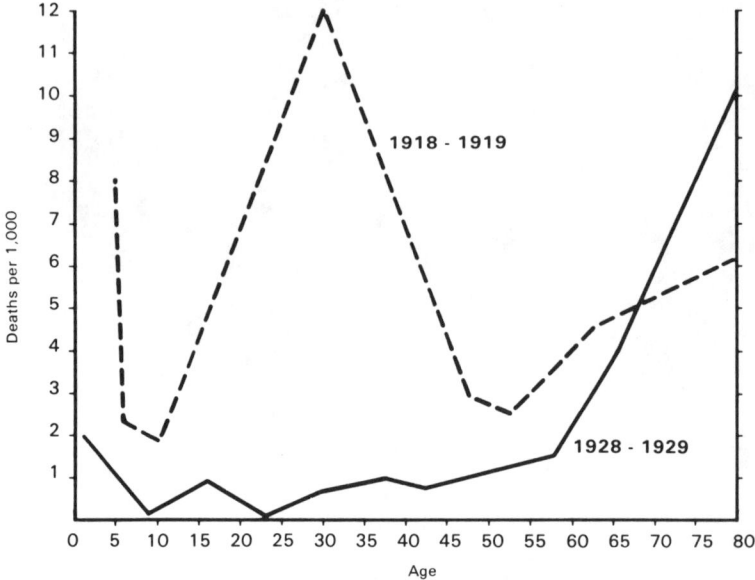

Figure 3.12. These comparative age-mortality graphs show just how different the episodes of 1918–20 and 1928–29 were.

The Depression Era: Continued Circulation and Discovery of the Virus

Public health records indicate that there were excess deaths from influenza-pneumonia nearly every winter during the Great Depression. The winters of greatest epidemic proportions in the United States were during 1932–33 and 1936–37.[54] Wintertime epidemics varied by year of occurrence in other parts of the world, but the prevailing strains during the 1930s were closely related; the relationships were known because influenza viruses were clearly identified as the cause of the disease in the early 1930s. Age-mortality profiles provided by Collins and his colleagues support the contention that the viruses found during the 1930s were more similar to the 1928–29 strain than to that of 1918–20.[55] Furthermore, virological discoveries during the Depression era led to conclusions that the Great Pandemic was caused by the swine influenza virus discovered in 1931.[56]

Geographical reconstructions of diffusion pathways during the 1930s also tend to suggest that there was some genetic drift over time, but no major shifts took place. For example, temporal mapping of peak mortality by regions by the Public Health Service during the first half of that decade indicated a rather slow movement of the disease around the country over a period of several years.[57] During the winter of 1930–31, mortality peaked first within the central southwest parts of the country and then all along the East Coast. During the following winter, the major epicenters were in the Mountain and central northwest regions, and by the 1932–33 epidemic season influenza was widespread. As the disease waned after the epidemic, early reporting foci had shifted to the East Coast once again by the winter of 1934–35.

In the early 1930s the initial discoveries of influenza viruses were made. Before 1931, when Richard Shope identified the virus that was causing influenza in swine in the United States,[58] it had long been thought that influenza in humans and animals was caused by viruses. This was the first absolute proof. Shope's discoveries were particularly important because influenza in swine was also a severe problem during the Great Pandemic, and some connection between the human and animal forms of the disease had been suspected for some time. During the 1930s, many actually believed that the human form of influenza experienced during World War I eventually moved to hogs to become an established disease.[59]

Meanwhile, the first clear evidence of human influenza viruses was produced by a British research team in 1933.[60] After repeated experiments with laboratory animals, Smith, Andrewes, and Laidlaw, with the assistance of Stuart-Harris, successfully transferred and isolated a virus that became known as "W.S." Soon after that, viruses known as "PR8" (from Puerto Rico) and "Phila" were identified by Francis and others in the United States.[61] In 1935, Burnet isolated a human influenza virus in Australia.[62]

Further laboratory studies of viruses during the 1930s revealed some interesting features of the agents. International comparisons initially led to the conclusion that viruses isolated in widespread locations were similar in structure.[63] However, another, different type of influenza virus was then discovered. The first broad group became known as Type "A" and the other, less common, as Type "B." At that time the swine influenza virus was recognized as yet another distinct entity. Still, as researchers continued to test for levels of immunity in search of an effective influenza vaccine, they found high levels of immunity to swine flu among persons who were old enough to have been around during the Great Pandemic and almost no immunity against that virus among those who had been born after 1920.

The epidemic of 1932–33 had provided sufficient quantities of virus around the world to assist in major discoveries. Progress continued throughout the 1930s, and it was just a matter of time until a vaccine would be developed. However, the mystery of the extreme virulence of the Great Pandemic remained unsolved.

Notes

1. Warren T. Vaughn, *Influenza: An Epidemiologic Study*. (Baltimore: American Journal of Hygiene, Monograph Series, No. 1, July, 1921), p. 2.
2. C. H. Stuart-Harris, "Influenza," in Walter R. Belt, ed., *The History and Conquest of Common Diseases* (Norman: University of Oklahoma Press, 1954), pp. 71–83.
3. Selwyn D. Collins, *Long-Time Trends in Illness and Medical Care* (Washington, D.C.: U.S. Department of Health, Education and Welfare, Public Health Service, Public Health Monograph No. 48, 1957).
4. Alfred Stengel, "The Influenza Epidemics of 1889 and 1918," *The Medical Clinics of North America* 2 (1918), pp. 645–69.
5. Edwin O. Kilbourne, "The Influenza Viruses and Influenza: An Introduction," in Kilbourne, ed. *The Influenza Viruses and Influenza* (New York: Academic Press, 1975).
6. F. M. Burnet and Ellen Clark, *Influenza: A Survey of the Last 50 Years in the Light of Modern Work on the Virus of Epidemic Influenza* (Melbourne: Macmillan, 1942), chap. 5.
7. Vaughn, *Influenza*, pp. 14–20.
8. Collins, *Long-Time Trends in Illness*, and Burnet and Clark, *Influenza*.
9. John H. Walters, "Influenza 1918: The Contemporary Perspective," *Bulletin, New York Academy of Medicine* 54 (1978), pp. 855–64.
10. Clifford A. Gill, *The Genesis of Epidemics and the Natural History of Disease* (New York: William Wood, 1928), chap. 15.
11. Edwin O. Jordan, *Epidemic Influenza: A Survey* (Chicago: American Medical Association, 1927), pp. 118–27.
12. Vaughn, *Influenza*, pp. 117–20.
13. Gill, *Genesis of Epidemics*, chap. 16.
14. Alfred W. Crosby, *Epidemic and Peace, 1918* (Westport, Conn.: Greenwood Press, 1976), chap. 1.
15. Idem, "The Influenza Pandemic of 1918," in June E. Osborn, *History, Science and Politics: Influenza in America* (New York: Prodist, 1977), pp. 5–9.
16. Burnet and Clark, *Influenza*, pp. 69–75.
17. Crosby, *Epidemic and Peace*, chap. 2.
18. Vaughn, *Influenza*, p. 68.
19. Jordan, *Epidemic Influenza*, p. 96.
20. Crosby, *Epidemic and Peace*, p. 25.
21. Ibid., p. 26.
22. Vaughn, *Influenza*, p. 68.
23. K. D. Patterson and Gerald F. Pyle. "The Diffusion of Influenza in Sub-Saharan Africa During the 1918–1919 Pandemic," *Social Science and Medicine* 17 (1983), pp. 1299–1307.
24. Gill, *Genesis of Epidemics*, chap. 16.
25. Vaughn, *Influenza*, pp. 65–70.
26. Crosby, *Epidemic and Peace*, p. 29.
27. Stuart-Harris, "Influenza."
28. Jay P. Sanford, "Influenza: Consideration of Pandemics," *Advances in Internal Medicine* 35 (1969), pp. 419–53; and Thomas Parran, "Pandemic Influenza," *Medical Annals of the District of Columbia* 12 (1943), pp. 425–27.
29. Selwyn D. Collins and Josephine Lehmann, "Trends and Epidemics of Influenza and Pneumonia, 1918–1951," *Public Health Reports* 46 (1951), pp. 1487–1516.
30. William H. Davis, "The Influenza Epidemic as Shown in the Weekly Health Index," *American Journal of Public Health* 9 (1919), pp. 50–61.
31. Edgar Sydenstricker, "Preliminary Statistics of the Influenza Epidemic," *Public Health Reports* 33 (December 27, 1918), pp. 2305–21.
32. Crosby, *Epidemic and Peace*, chap. 5.
33. Jordan, *Epidemic Influenza*, p. 119.
34. Sydenstricker, "Preliminary Statistics of the Influenza Epidemic," p. 2311.

35. Extensive files are kept in the National Archives on the 1918–20 pandemic, but as of April 1984, Sydenstricker's files on 376 cities were not among them.
36. Jordan, *Epidemic Influenza,* pp. 125–41.
37. Raymond Pearl, "Future Data on the Correlation of Explosiveness of Outbreak of the 1918 Epidemic," *Public Health Reports* 36 (February 18, 1921), pp. 273–98.
38. Idem, "On Certain General Statistical Aspects of the 1918 Epidemic in American Cities," *Public Health Reports* 34 (August 8, 1919), pp. 1743–75.
39. Crosby, *Epidemic and Peace,* chap. 6.
40. U.S. Public Health Service, *Public Health Reports* 34 (February 7, 1919), pp. 226–29.
41. W. H. Frost and Edgar Sydenstricker, "Influenza in Maryland: Preliminary Statistics of Certain Localities," *Public Health Reports* 34 (March 14, 1919), pp. 491–505.
42. C. E. A. Winslow and J. F. Rogers, "Statistics of the 1918 Epidemic of Influenza in Connecticut," *Journal of Infectious Diseases* 26 (1920), pp. 185–216.
43. Ibid., p. 214.
44. John Dill Robertson and Gottfried Koehler, "Preliminary Report on the Influenza Epidemic in Chicago," *American Journal of Public Health* 8 (1918), pp. 851–56.
45. Edwin O. Jordan, Dudley B. Reed, and E. B. Fink, "Influenza in Three Chicago Groups," *Journal of Infectious Diseases* 25 (1919), pp. 74–95.
46. D. G. Stine, "A Comparison of the Influenza Epidemic of 1918 with that of 1920 at the University of Missouri," *Journal of the Missouri State Medical Association* 18 (1921), pp. 117–123.
47. Ibid., p. 120.
48. Selwyn D. Collins, W. H. Frost, Mary Gover, and Edgar Sydenstricker, "Mortality from Influenza and Pneumonia in 50 Large Cities of the United States, 1910–1929," *Public Health Reports* 45 (September 26, 1930), pp. 2277–2328.
49. Frank M. Burnet and David O. White, *The Natural History of Infectious Diseases* (Cambridge: Cambridge University Press, 1972), pp. 202–12.
50. Collins, *Long-Time Trends in Illness.*
51. Collins and Lehmann, "Trends and Epidemics."
52. Idem, *Excess Deaths from Influenza and Pneumonia and from Important Chronic Diseases during Epidemic Periods, 1918–1951* (Washington, D.C.: U.S. Public Health Service, Public Health Monograph No. 10, 1951).
53. Collins, *Long-Time Trends in Illness.*
54. Collins and Lehmann, *Excess Deaths from Influenza.*
55. Ibid.
56. Richard E. Shope, "The Incidence of Neutralizing Antibodies for Swine Influenza Virus in the Sera of Human Beings of Different Ages," *Journal of Experimental Medicine* 63 (1936), pp. 669–84.
57. Selwyn D. Collins and Mary Gover, "Influenza and Pneumonia Mortality in a Group of about 95 cities in the United States during Four Minor Epidemics, 1930–35, With a Summary for 1920–35," *Public Health Reports* 50 (November 29, 1935), pp. 1668–89.
58. Richard E. Shope, "Swine Influenza," *Journal of Experimental Medicine* 54 (1931), pp. 373–85.
59. C. H. Andrewes, "Thoughts on the Origin of Influenza Epidemics," *Proceedings, Royal Society of Medicine* 36 (1942), pp. 1–10.
60. Wilson Smith, C. H. Andrewes, and P. P. Laidlaw, "A Virus Obtained from Influenza Patients," *Lancet* (July 8, 1933), pp. 66–68.
61. Thomas Francis, Jr., "Epidemiological Studies in Influenza," *American Journal of Public Health* 27 (1937), pp. 211–25.
62. F. M. Burnet, "Influenza Virus Isolated from an Australian Epidemic," *Medical Journal of Australia* (September 9, 1935), pp. 651–53.
63. T. P. Magill and Thomas Francis, Jr., "Antigenic Differences in Strains of Human Influenza Virus," *Proceedings, Society of Experimental Biology and Medicine* 35 (1935), pp. 463–66.

4

Influenza Patterns in the 1940s

Influenza-diffusion patterns during and immediately after World War II were characterized by both multiepicenter eruptions during various winters and the possible entry of a different strain of the disease into the United States during the late 1940s. Influenza was responsible for an untold number of wintertime deaths during the Great Depression, and a particularly bad epidemic occurred during the winter of 1936–37.[1] Excessive wintertime influenza deaths ushered in the 1940s, and the disease decreased in intensity for three seasons, only to increase again during the winter of 1943–44. That epidemic was caused by a strain of influenza closely related to those identified in the 1930s, and it was therefore not surprising to find similar geographical patterns of influenza diffusion. A vaccine had also been developed to counteract the prevailing strain of influenza during the early 1940s, but it seemed to have little effect on the particular strain of influenza that caused an epidemic during the winter of 1947–48. Also, the 1947 strain moved through the country somewhat differently than the 1943–44 strain.

Influenza reports and studies from the 1940s indicated for more than three decades that the two major strains of the 1940s were indeed sufficiently different to be considered separate types. Various designations were used in making the distinction. For example, the earlier form was considered "A" and the later either "A1" or "A-prime."[2] Later, with increased awareness of the relationship between hemagglutinin and neuraminidase spikes, the designations H0N1 and H1N1 were also used.[3] Since it was strongly suspected that "swine flu" had caused the Great Pandemic of 1918–20, the designation Hsw1N1 was used to make a further distinction. Recent reexaminations of the virology of influenza during the 1940s have concluded that all three of these viral types are more closely related to each other than to strains that emerged in the 1950s and 1960s.[4]

This chapter is adapted from Gerald F. Pyle, "Geographical Perspectives on Influenza Diffusion: The United States in the 1940's," in Melinda S. Meade, ed., *Conceptual and Methodological Issues in Medical Geography* (Chapel Hill: University of North Carolina, Department of Geography, Studies in Geography No. 15, 1980), pp. 222–49.

In light of these conclusions, an examination of the geographical epidemiology of the most important influenza epidemics in the 1940s with comparisons with earlier episodes might be of assistance in understanding similarities and differences among strains. Given the ever-present possibility that the geography of different strains also varies, the major purpose of this chapter is to offer a spatial comparison of the epidemics of 1943–44 and 1947–48 so that some of the variable notions about the diffusion of influenza can be tested.

The Early 1940s

Within a decade of the clear identification of the influenza virus, leading scientists, including Francis, Lennette, Hirst, Rickard, Horstfall, and others, had made tremendous strides with regard to the specification and nomenclature of various types of virus,[5,6] the etiology of epidemic influenza,[7] and factors contributing to influenza resistance.[8] Such possibilities as the recycling of different strains in time and cocirculation were also beginning to be considered, and vaccines were being perfected. In addition, Collins and his co-workers at the Public Health Service continued to monitor influenza patterns and apply various forms of statistical analysis.[9] The system of voluntary reporting of influenza-pneumonia mortality from various urban centers that had begun during the Great Pandemic continued into the 1940s. As some cities entered the system over time and others dropped out, anywhere from 80 to 100 urban areas can be accounted for during the 1940s with regard to weekly reporting of influenza deaths. In addition, influenza morbidity during the epidemic of 1943–44 was reported weekly.[10]

Some general accounts of the geography of influenza were also attempted in the early 1940s. For example, the Public Health Service reported that during the 1940–41 season, high mortality rates were initially reported in the Mountain and Pacific regions, and the disease then may have spread rapidly into the southern parts of the country.[11] This activity is presumed to have been due to the prevailing type A virus, and it was probably the continued circulation of the same agent that resulted in excessive mortality during the previous winter. After influenza had apparently spread to the Southeast, certain Mid-Atlantic, northeastern, and Great Lakes areas also reached the "excess mortality" level. It is difficult to ascertain whether this activity could truly have been considered an epidemic at that time, but it would be today. Collins did consider this to be the sixteenth such epidemic since the pandemic of 1918–20. He also wrote that excessive deaths credited primarily to the influenza-pneumonia epidemics of the early 1940s were smaller in magnitude than most of those of the 1930s.[12] A major feature that stands out about this early 1940s activity is that points of origin appear to be more or less "indigenous," and they may in fact have been part of continued cyclical activity. What is important about this part of the 1940s is that research in understanding the nature of viruses had increased, and scientists began to understand more clearly the nature of hemagglutination.[13] The early 1940s experienced relatively mild influenza activity compared to the 1930s, but they were followed by a major epidemic that was thought to have begun during the early part of the 1943–44 winter season, with a presumed national peak on December 29, 1943.

The 1943–44 Epidemic

When the death rates attributed to influenza-pneumonia are compared for each winter of the 1940s, the 1943–44 season clearly stands out as having had the most severe epidemic. Furthermore, strong evidence indicates that the epidemic was not caused by a "new" virus. Instead, it seems to have been perpetuated by the continued circulation of a prevailing strain. As with influenza epidemics before and after, the one that occurred during the winter of 1943–44 was initiated by a springtime flare-up, but it was not substantial. Accounts at that time indicate that from December 1941 through March 1943 the number of reported cases of influenza-pneumonia mortality varied little from the five-year median used for previous corresponding months.[14] However, by December 1943 it was clear that the country was in the midst of yet another influenza epidemic. One possible questionable indication came from morbidity reports for cities where reporting was discontinued during the 1970s and 1980s. During this period, and perhaps because of wartime conditions and the discovery of influenza among many service people, morbidity reporting from some cities increased drastically during December 1943 and January 1944.[15] Figure 4.1 shows these increases for New York City; Columbus, Ohio; Charleston, South Carolina; Birmingham, Alabama; and San Francisco and Los Angeles. The horizontal scales used for the morbidity reports ("cases") in Figure 4.1 begin with the first week of July 1943. In fact, it is common in many analyses of influenza to start measuring during the summer, when there are low levels of activity. One of the major problems associated with morbidity reporting shows up particularly with the information from San Francisco. Morbidity reporting virtually did not exist for several months; then, perhaps with the realization of a problem during the winter, cases suddenly increased drastically.

When Collins analyzed the 1943–44 epidemic a year later, he stated

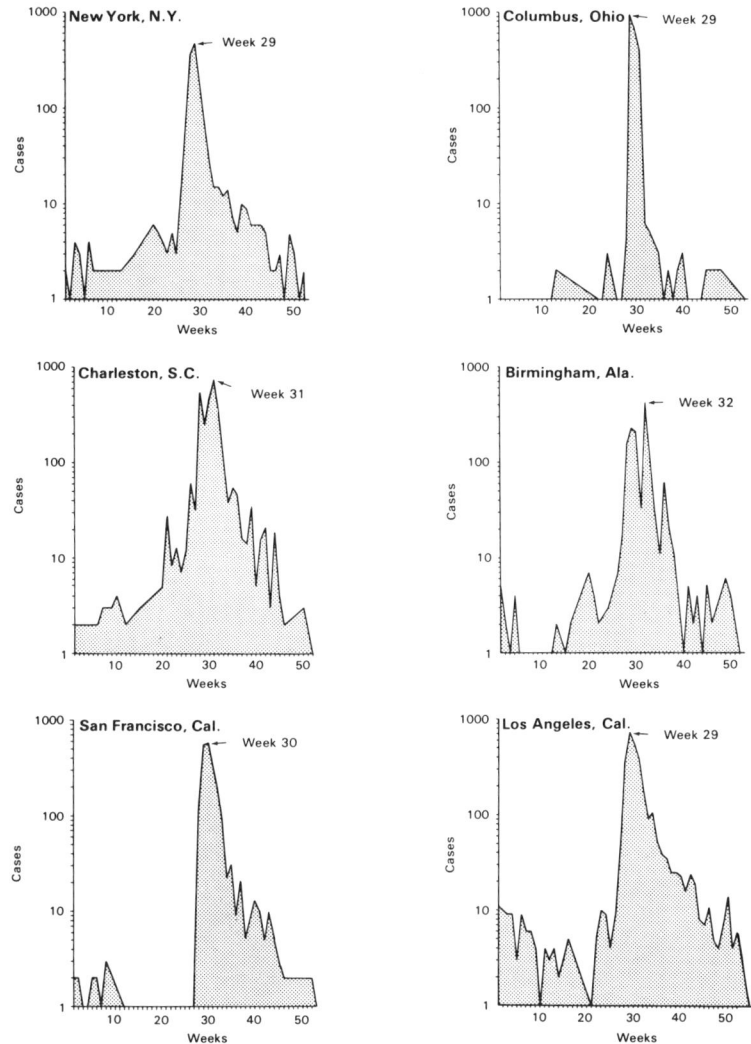

Figure 4.1. Morbidity reporting from selected cities during the winter of 1943–44. Reading along each *x*-axis, the first week begins in July.

that the number of deaths may in fact have been fewer than those of the 1936–37 and 1932–33 epidemics, which in turn were smaller than those of the 1928–29 and 1926 epidemics.[16] Also, some data for the 1943–44 epidemic from a United States Census Bureau report consist of a 10 percent mortality sample from all states, and that information indicated that the rate may have been actually higher than reported by the Public Health Service.[17] In addition, Collins based his analysis of specific rates on information from 90 cities, thus adding an urban bias to his results.

Epidemiological researchers continued to develop a better understanding of the temporal periodicity and age-cohort distributions on the basis of the 1943–44 epidemic. With regard to age cohorts, Public Health Service reports showed how the mortality "bulge" in the cohort distribution had shifted from the 20-to-40-year-old group in the early 1920s to the elderly by 1943–44. In fact, that shift had shown up by 1928, and it continued into the 1930s and 1940s.[18] Still, these conclusions were reached using the Collins "excess mortality" measure based on any previous five years (Chapter 3). When proportions of deaths by given cohorts are examined by specific years, there was a fairly substantial proportion of mortality among those from 5 to 14 years old during the winter of 1943–44.[19] Perhaps the Depression and World War II conditions of economic austerity, combined with exposure to a variety of childhood diseases, led to overall lowered resistance to influenza within that cohort.

On the matter of periodicity from one year to the next, a report two years later from the Commission on Influenza established in 1943 stated:

> The 16 widespread epidemics of influenza which have occurred in the United States between 1920 and 1944 can be accounted for on the basis of two specific recurrent infections. Influenza A appears to have a cycle of two to three years and influenza B of four to six years. There is no indication that other influenza viruses have caused widespread epidemics in the country in the past 25 years. On the basis of this information, the probability of occurrence of future epidemics within certain time limits has been forecast. It has been suggested that the balance between immune and susceptible individuals in the population is the dominant factor which determines the occurrence of influenza epidemics.[20]

These findings indicate that at that time attempts were made to identify regular cycles of two types of influenza similar to the two kinds of measles. Events during the next forty years proved that influenza cycles are indeed more complicated.

Some Statistical and Geographical Characteristics of the 1943–44 Epidemic

Statistical and cartographic comparisons of 1943–44 influenza-mortality data help in determining the characteristics of that epidemic.[21] Initially, it is useful to compare the various influenza seasons of the 1940s in the context of logistic distributions similar to those used in studying spatial diffusion in general. Figure 4.2 compares the various seasons. For these comparisons on a "national" basis, Week 1 is considered as the first week of July for any given annual cycle, and

Week 52 is approximately the last week in June of the next year. Using this method of comparison, it is clear that the 1943–44 epidemic had a faster rate of temporal increase than any of the other seasons of influenza activity during that decade. Death rates per 100,000 were also higher during the 1943–44 epidemic. The "national" totals used to construct the comparisons in Figure 4.2 are based on reports from approximately 77 cities that offered information consistently during the 1940s and were within statistical confidence limits. These cumulative-frequency distributions based on death rates are a useful way to determine the velocity of influenza diffusion. However, they apply only to the statistical aggregate of the cities.

To understand spatiotemporal variations at various geographic points, it is useful to calculate such a statistical distribution for each

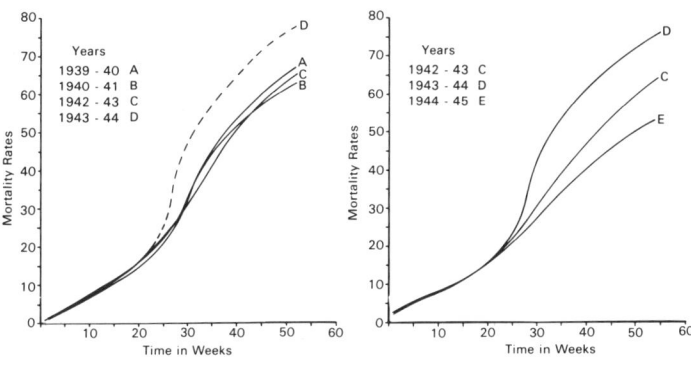

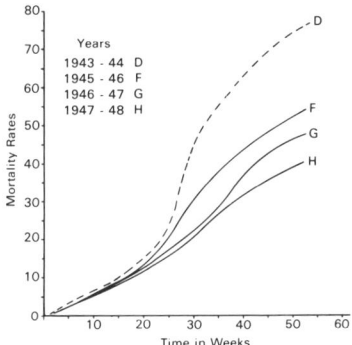

Figure 4.2. Epidemic curves showing cumulative influenza mortality during selected 1940s winters. In each instance, the *x*-axis originates during the first week of July.

point. This was accomplished for the group of cities that were aggregated to the national totals, and approximately 66 of those cities reported enough statistically significant distributions to demonstrate a meaningful logistic shape during the 1943–44 epidemic. As noted in Chapter 1, reporting for any annual influenza cycle running from the first of July of one year to the thirtieth of June of the next year may not be an accurate measure of disease activity. For some cities, influenza activity may decline at a more rapid rate in the spring than in other cities. In addition, increases in influenza-mortality reporting may start as early as June and continue to increase in some places, while in others, increases may not start until September and October.

Given this phenomenon, a more detailed examination of the spring influenza activity in 1943 (previously presumed to be the end part of a nonepidemic year) reveals that in many places there was somewhat higher-than-normal springtime reporting of influenza mortality. This oscillation consisted of a December-to-January wintertime peaking of influenza-pneumonia mortality, a decline in rates in late winter or early spring, and then increased spring activity followed by a major decline. Again, the pertinent issue to be addressed when examining this sort of phenomenon is whether or not it may be a form of spring seeding. If so, is it in fact the same kind of "A" virus that has been circulating within the United States for several decades? After having examined the spring 1943 phenomenon, it is contended here that some viral drift occurred, but it was not a major shift. In most instances a December-to-January "normal" influenza peak was noted, followed by decreases and then some increased springtime reporting. This increase, when taken in the context of influenza-diffusion theory, is assumed to be a form of "drift seeding" followed by decreases during the spring of 1943 and then rapid autumn increases leading to peaking either during December 1943 or January 1944, the previously identified winter of the epidemic.

Evidence of the directions of springtime spread in 1943 is presented in the two maps in Figure 4.3. Parts of the country that indicated earliest "drift seeding" were the Texas and Louisiana Gulf Coast, the Upper Mississippi Valley, and a large section of the interior of the country extending from Denver to Omaha. Another diffusion pathway from Denver to Kansas City to Omaha, Topeka, and Wichita can be identified. Yet another was from Houston and Galveston to Shreveport, New Orleans, Little Rock, and Dallas (Fig. 4.3, Spring). The spread was somewhat rapid, with large parts of the central United States being encompassed within a two-month period. There was also some diffusion southward along the Pacific coast, as well as movement from the Mississippi Valley into the Ohio–Michigan–Pennsylvania area. In New England, Bridgeport and Providence showed early seeding. The disease then erupted in Boston, Hartford, New Haven, Springfield, Portland, and Fall River. In general, Figure 4.3 shows the postulated movement of "clinical fronts" due to probable seeding.

The seeding waned, as expected, to be followed by outbreaks of the major wave of the epidemic during the late summer and fall of 1943 (Fig. 4.3, Autumn). The maps in Figure 4.4 detail the earlier and later

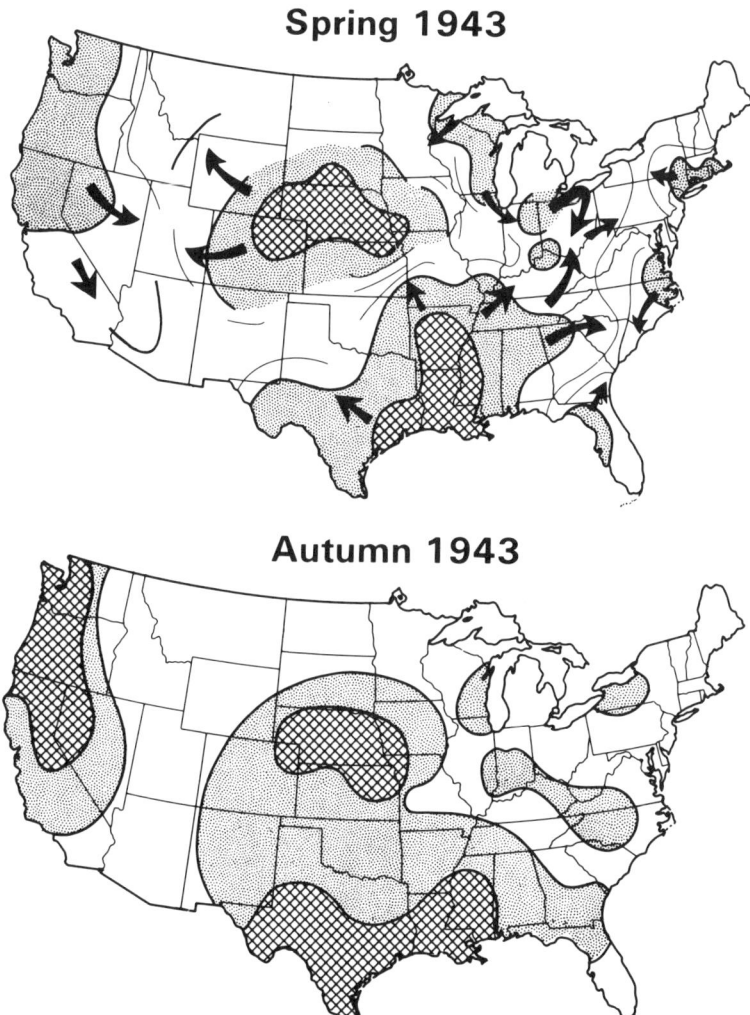

Spring 1943

Autumn 1943

Figure 4.3. These maps show how some, but not all, of the early influenza-outbreak centers during the spring of 1943 were also epicenters during the autumn of that year.

stages of the main wave of the epidemic. Also indicated are areas with the earliest outbreaks at the beginning of the epidemic, essentially in the same parts of the country demonstrating the earliest spring seeding. By the time the epidemic peaked (about December 29, 1943), most of the remainder of the country was accounted for, as shown in Figure 4.5. Some of the earliest peaking occurred in areas that were adjacent to the initial outbreaks during the presumed seeding process. To determine the possibility of hierarchical effects, various cumulative percentiles of individual cities were tested on a temporal scale against city size. No significant fit was accomplished other than with the numbers of cases expected in accordance with city size. It can therefore be stated that the 1943–44 influenza epidemic in the United States had the following characteristics:

1. It was not hierarchical with respect to city size and outward diffusion.
2. The epidemic can be considered multinodal, with earliest outbreaks in the central parts of the country, followed by coastal areas.
3. If some form of seeding did indeed take place, then this information could in fact be used to predict areas of early outbreak during the fall and winter of 1943.
4. Forms of diffusion appeared to be contagious in nature, probably demonstrating both fairly long-distance linear as well as radial patterns, as can be seen in Figures 4.4 and 4.5.

In retrospect, in the context of current influenza virus nomenclature, the 1943–44 epidemic is now considered to be due to some variants of H1N1. Yet, a vaccine that had been developed prior to that epidemic proved to be ineffective during a subsequent episode. This raises the question as to whether or not the subsequent epidemic consisted of the introduction of a truly different viral strain. At least most influenza authorities now believe that the 1943–44 epidemic was not caused by a new strain. This latter contention is given some support by an analysis of the nature of the outbreak and geographical diffusion of the disease. It was introduced into the country in major seaport cities, in larger urban centers, or in those areas that carried inordinately large amounts of passenger-train traffic. It was probably caused by a variant of a prevailing virus endemic to the United States.

Influenza in the Late 1940s: A New Strain?

The epidemic of 1947–48 is actually better documented than that of 1943–44 even though, fortunately, it was instrumental in far fewer deaths in the United States. According to Francis, Salk, and Quilligan, the 1947–48 epidemic was expected on the basis of accumulated experience.[22] In fact, the epidemic was different from previous outbreaks during the 1940s in several respects:

1. The epidemic was anticipated in advance.
2. Some vaccination attempts were underway during the epidemic.
3. The epidemic was probably of extraneous origin; that is, its pattern may have been different from that explained as the continued oscillation of an existing strain.
4. In spite of lower mortality rates, it was ultimately more widespread throughout the country.
5. It was not as severe in terms of mortality as the 1943–44 epidemic.
6. The epidemic was followed in several subsequent seasons by increases in influenza B activity.

Between October 22 and November 2, 1946, in anticipation of an epidemic because of information from Europe, more than 10,000 University of Michigan students voluntarily received vaccinations, and another group of nearly 8,000 not receiving the vaccine were used in statistical comparisons.[23] A new strain had presumably entered the country from extraneous sources, but illness levels were approximately the same in vaccinated versus nonvaccinated students. One problem seems to be that the vaccine may have been administered prior to the arrival of a new or different strain of influenza. Accounts vary on when a different type of influenza entered the country. The virus now referred to as the 1947 strain (and sometimes the 1951 strain) was not really discovered until the spring of 1947.[24] Antibodies developed from viruses characteristic of previous epidemics appeared in students tested near the end of the epidemic, but new antibodies resulting from the arrival of a new strain were also discovered. In general, the vaccine developed to combat the earlier strain was not effective against the new strain.

Reported influenza-mortality data from various cities during the 1946–48 period compared with the 1942–44 period shows that 63 cities were statistically significant for both epidemics. Initially, comparisons of monthly reporting for the two epidemics were made for these cities. In more than 50 cities, a clearly discernible late-winter–early-spring troughing was noted, followed by spring peaking for both periods. There was an apparent lull in influenza activity prior to a minor peak appearing, according to Collins, as late as March 16, 1947.[25] Figures 4.6 and 4.7 depict monthly comparisons for selected cities in different parts of the United States during the two epidemics. These comparisons indicate how the 1943–44 epidemic was indeed

September 1943

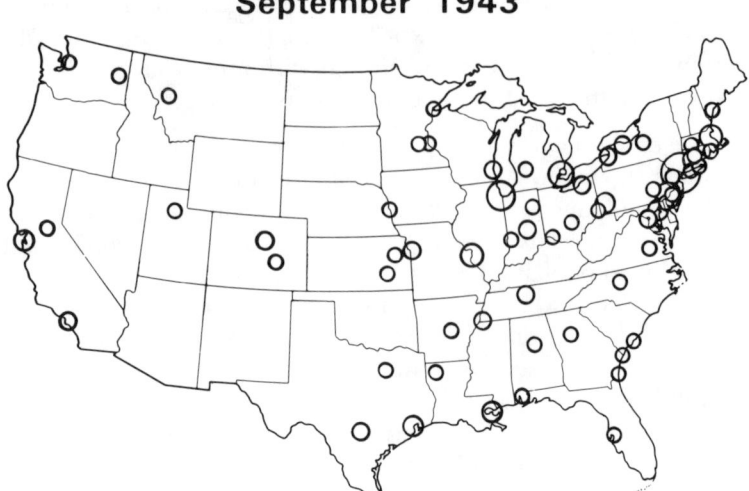

October 1943

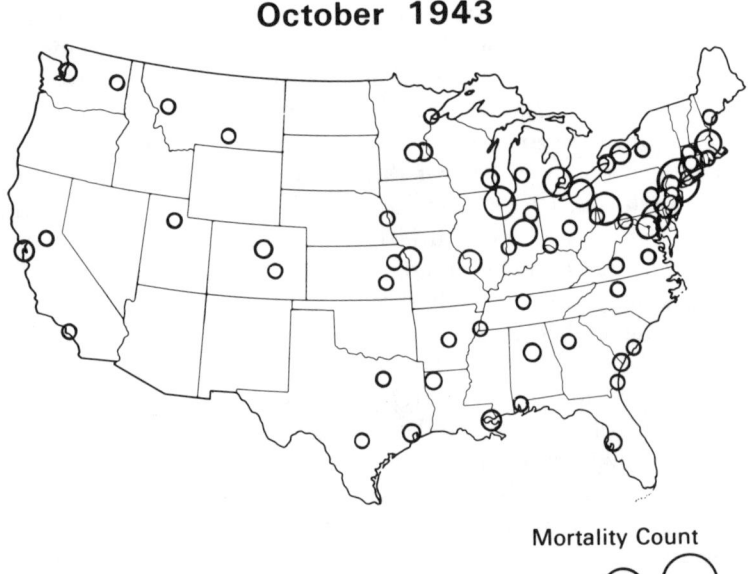

Mortality Count

10   75   250   1000

Figure 4.4. During the autumn of 1943, increases in influenza mortality were widespread.

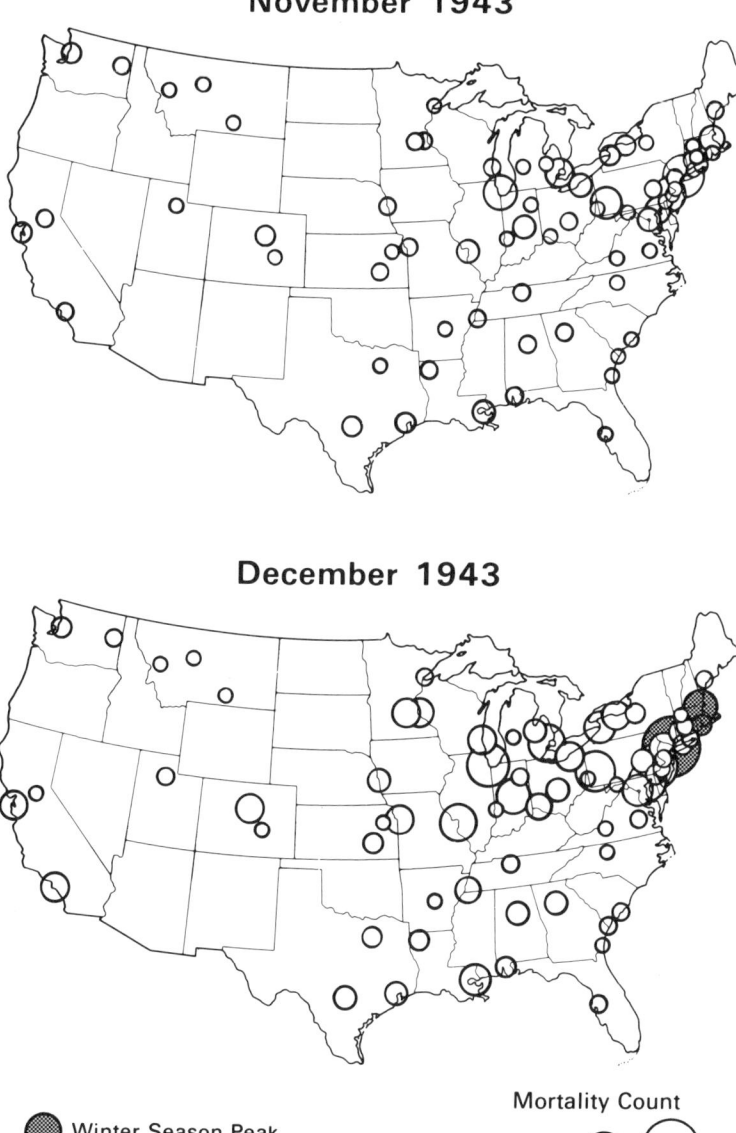

Figure 4.5. In spite of widespread endemic influenza in November and December 1943, cities did not begin to peak until December, and that happened first in New York City, Boston, and Providence.

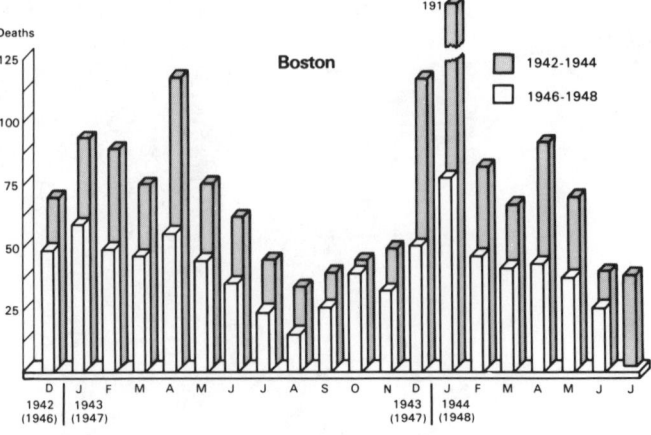

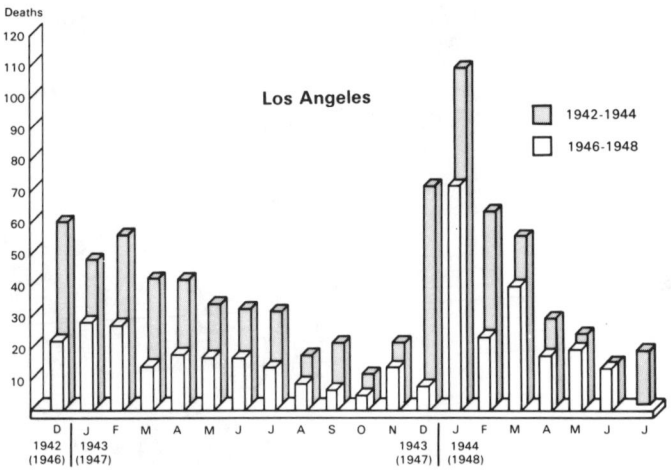

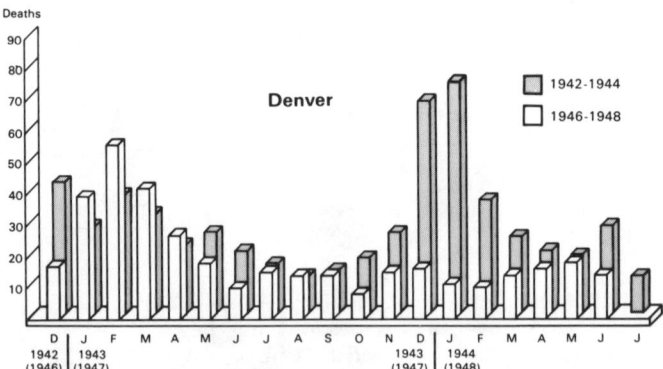

Figure 4.6. The mortality reporting from Boston, Los Angeles, and Denver for 1943–44 and 1947–48 shows the magnitude of both epidemics.

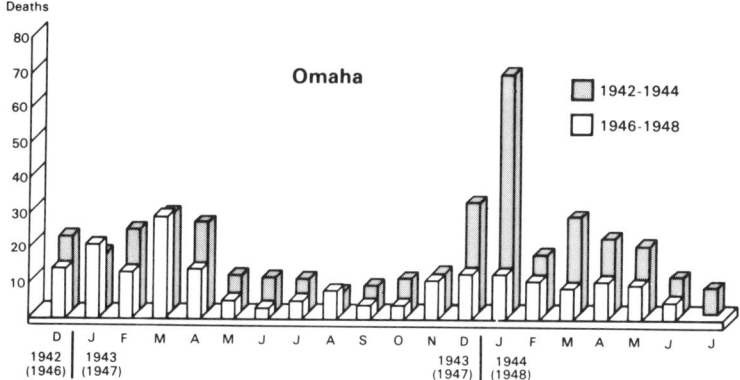

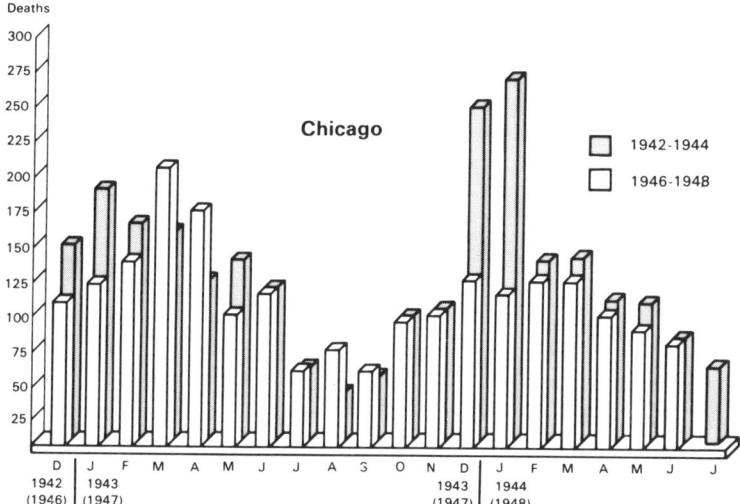

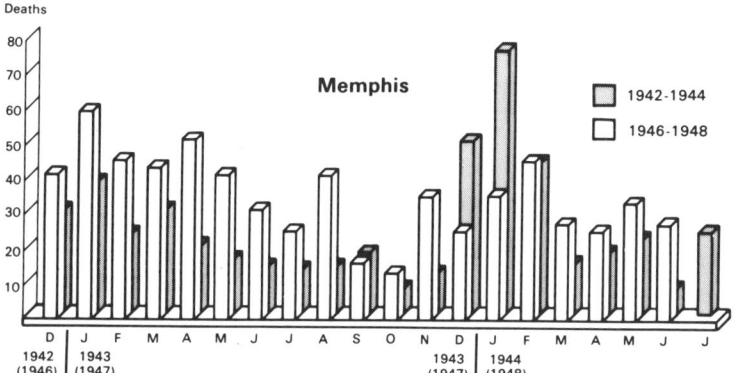

Figure 4.7. Influenza-mortality reporting from Omaha, Chicago, and Memphis during the epidemics of 1943–44 and 1947–48.

February 1947

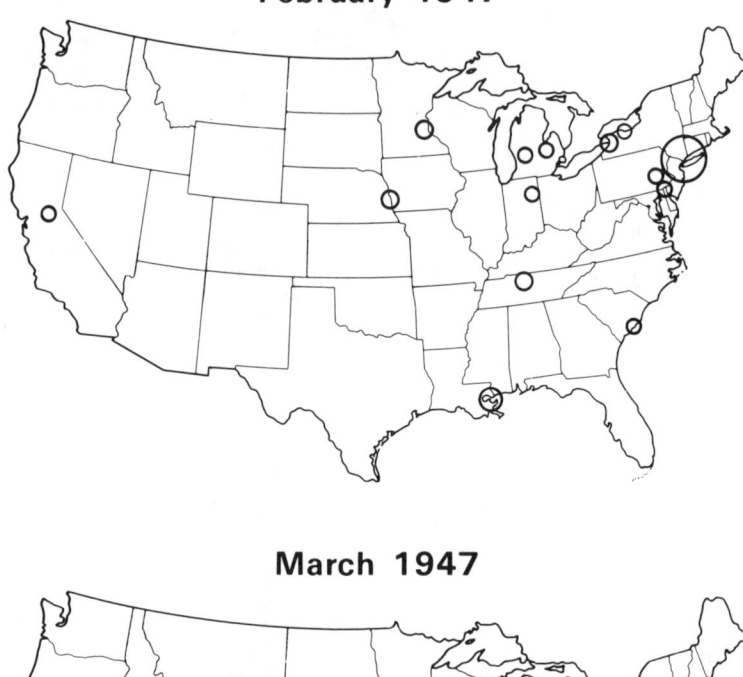

March 1947

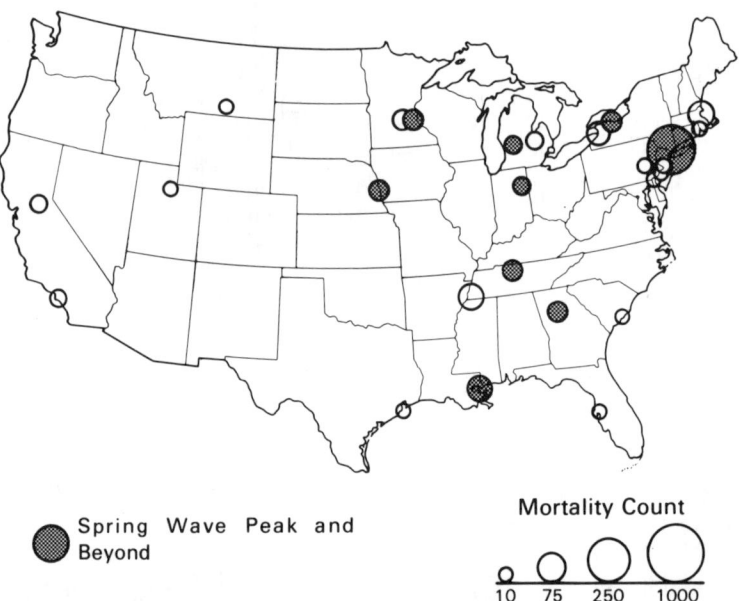

● Spring Wave Peak and Beyond

Mortality Count

○ ○ ○ ○
10   75   250   1000

Figure 4.8. Cities with unusually high springtime influenza activity during 1947. This kind of reporting also was done prior to previous and subsequent epidemics, yet the geographical pattern of wave peaking suggests endemic influenza because of the widespread reports.

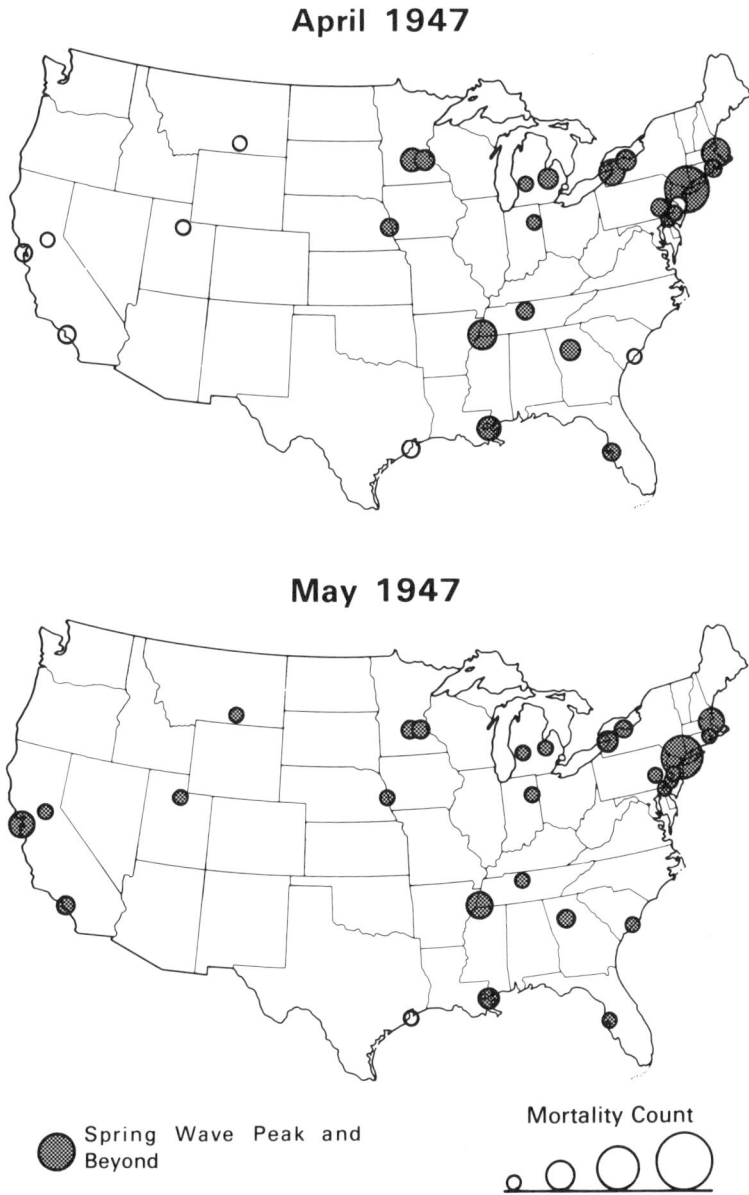

Figure 4.9. More widespread influenza peaking during the spring of 1947.

more severe in terms of mortality than that of the winter of 1947–48. A more detailed examination of temporal aspects of mortality also indicates that some form of drift seeding may have taken place during the spring of 1947, but influenza deaths never reached the proportions during the winter of 1947–48 that were obtained during the winter of 1943–44. In other words, drift was probably taking place, but the 1947 variant of influenza was far less virulent than the earlier form.

Reconstructed patterns of probable spatial diffusion also strongly suggest that viral drift may have continued through the summer of 1947 in the western Great Lakes area, as well as in parts of the eastern Great Lakes, parts of the Eastern Seaboard, Florida, the West Coast, and the Mississippi Delta. For example, there is some suggestion of penetration into the country from extraneous sources during February and March 1947 (Fig. 4.8), but outbreaks occurred in more interior parts of the country as well. The general tendency during March and April seems to have been characterized by a degree of diffusion from East to West (Fig. 4.9). Some influenza apparently spread radially from the points of origin. Once again, statistical testing did not uncover any strong hierarchial effects.

The disease then waned during the summer of 1947, but only for a short period. By July and August it had flared up again and spread from epicenters in Colorado, the Gulf Coast, the Midwest, and the Mid-Atlantic states. The patterns of spread shown in Figure 4.10 suggest that perhaps viral drift continued because areas infected during the spring of 1947 were affected once again in the late summer and early autumn. Moreover, that spread continued into the winter in a similar fashion. By November only a few cities had reached the fiftieth percentile (solid circles) of their wintertime distribution, and by December many places adjacent to the epicenters had reached that measure (Figs. 4.11 and 4.12). By January most cities in the traditional Manfacturing Belt had reached their midpoint,[26] and by February influenza had saturated most major cities.

Was the 1947 Virus Substantially Different?

The analysis in this chapter neither supports nor refutes the notion that the 1947–48 epidemic was caused by a virus of extraneous origin. Instead, it describes several interesting features concerning the reliability of reporting data, the measurement of lead and lag time in influenza diffusion, and differential rates of mortality and spread associated with drifting viruses. The use of aggregated-city-reporting data can now be considered of historical utility, but it is of little use

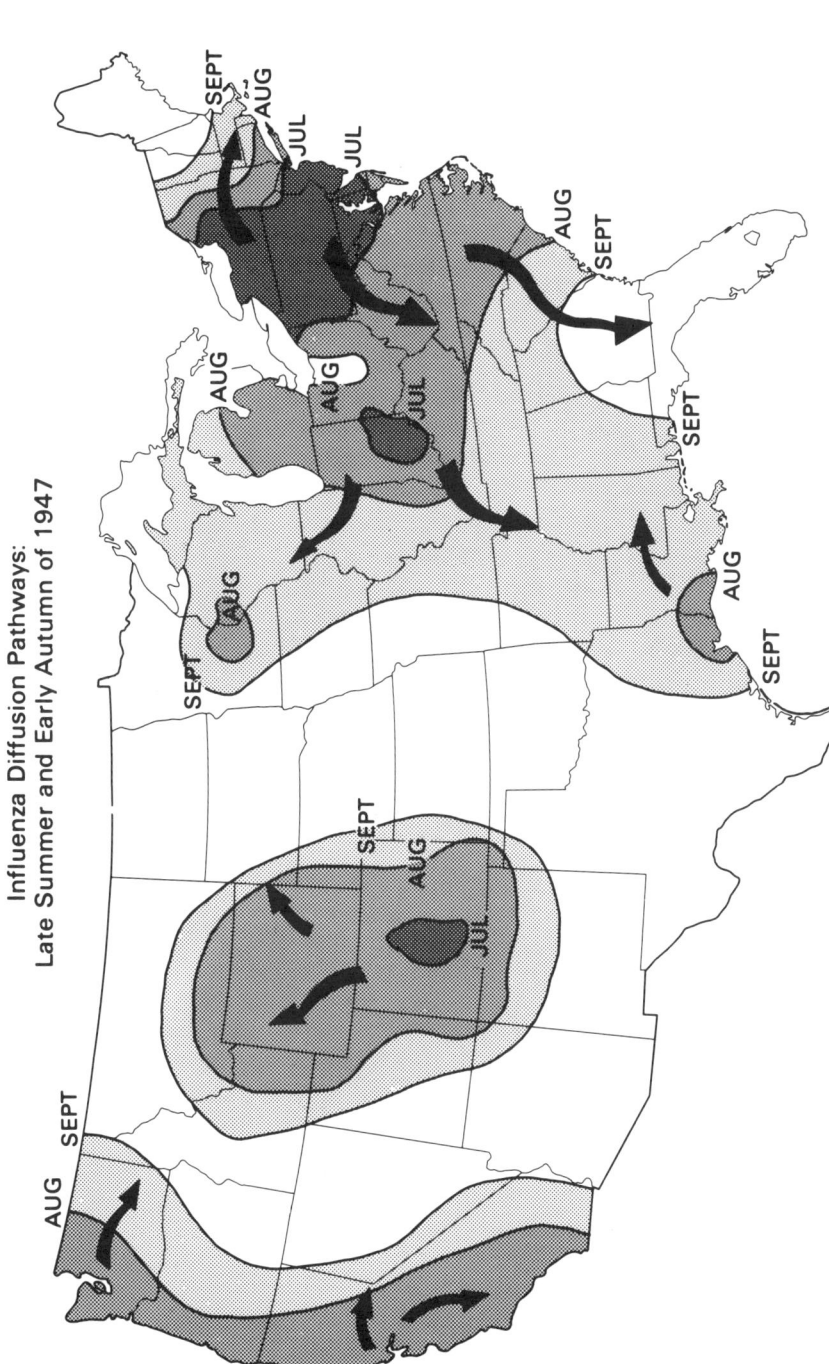

Influenza Diffusion Pathways:
Late Summer and Early Autumn of 1947

Figure 4.10. Outbreaks of influenza during early autumn 1947. The areas of earliest reporting were much more concentrated than during the spring of 1947, suggesting the entry of a new strain into the country.

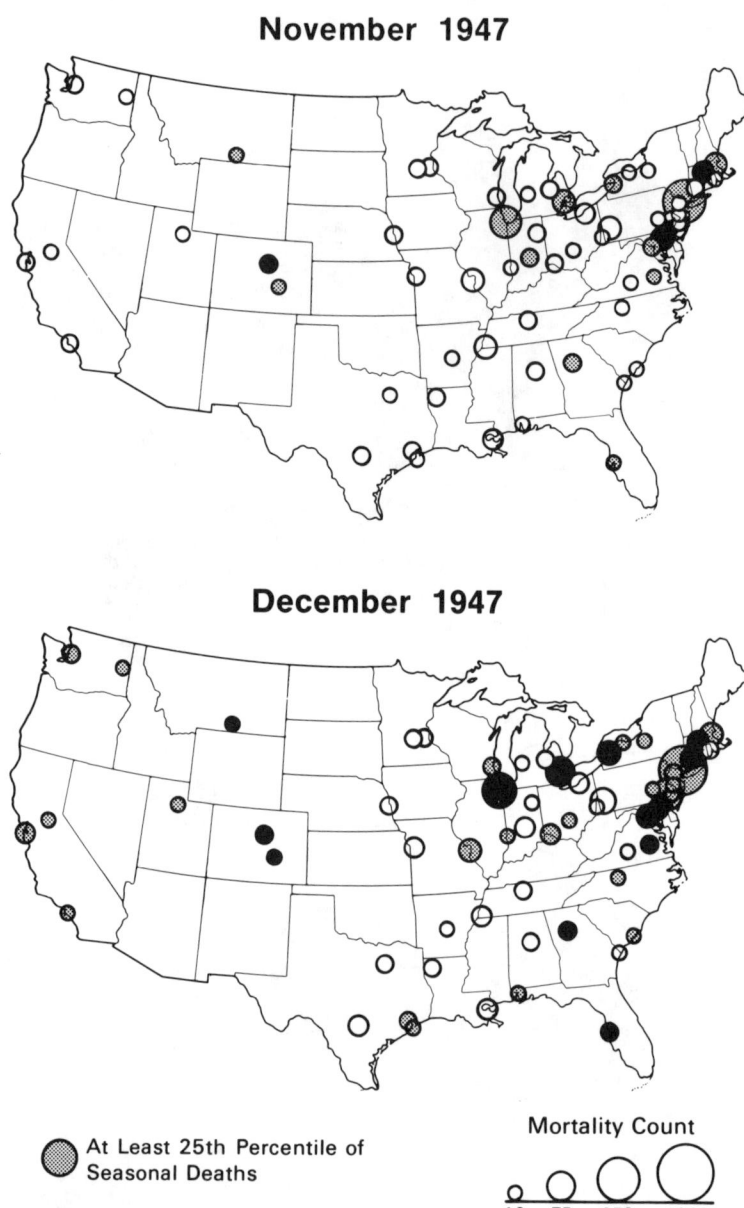

Figure 4.11. These maps show how the epidemic strain of influenza spread through urban areas during the autumn of 1947.

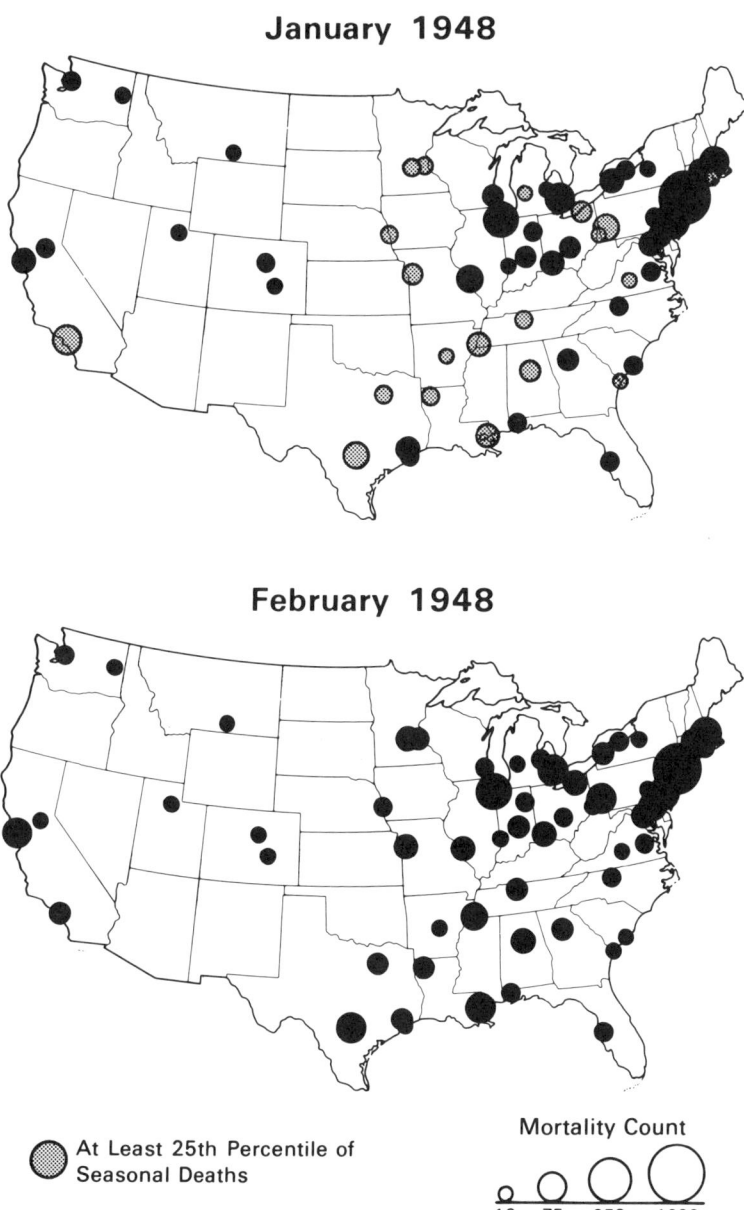

Figure 4.12. By January 1948, influenza had peaked within Manufacturing Belt cities, and by February the new strain had become firmly established.

with respect to surveillance and advance warning of the major introduction of new and possibly virulent strains. Cities must be measured
on an individual basis. Likewise, whether 70, 80, or 100 cities are used
as leading indicators of influenza activity, not all reporting can be
considered accurate because of a variety of reasons uncovered when
testing for statistical confidence. Conversely, it is possible through the
use of mortality reporting to gain sufficient insight into influenza
activity to develop more sophisticated methods of simulating possible
future epidemics. An intriguing aspect of this consideration is the
somewhat unexpected arrival once again of the H1N1 strain in the
late 1970s. According to Pereira, H1N1 (also referred to as A/USSR/
90/77) is a "historical" virus that surprisingly reemerged in late 1977.[27]
The World Health Organization was informed by the National Influenza Center of Moscow that this virus was isolated in different parts
of the Soviet Union in the late 1970s after having "disappeared" in
1957 (see Chapter 5). Additional investigations indicated that perhaps
the late-1970s virus had originated in China, spread through the
Soviet Union into Eastern and then Western Europe and on into
parts of the United States (see Chapter 7). Earlier, influenza researchers had also argued that the 1947 virus was of Oriental origin.
However, in light of 1980s conclusions that the epidemics of the
1970s, 1930s, and 1940s were really all caused by closely related
viruses, then there is just as much support for the argument that
genetic recombination in the form of drift and shift probably can take
place in North America. In conclusion, no one is really sure even
today where the epidemic of 1947–48 originated.

Notes

1. Mary Gover, "Influenza and Pneumonia Mortality in a Group of 90 Cities in the
   United States, August 1935–March 1943, with a summary for August 1920–March
   1943," U.S. Public Health Service, *Public Health Reports* 58 (July 9, 1943), pp. 1033–
   62; Selwyn D. Collins and Josephine Lehmann, "Trends and Epidemics of Influenza and Pneumonia, 1918–1951," *Public Health Reports* 66 (1951) pp. 1487–1516.
2. Thomas Francis, Jr., "Factors Conditioning Resistance to Epidemic Influenza," *The
   Harvey Lectures*, vol. 37 (New York: The Harvey Lecture Series, 1941), pp. 69–99;
   Thomas Francis, Jr., "On the Doctrine of Original Antigenic Sin," *Proceedings of the
   American Philosophical Society* 104 (1960), pp. 572–78.
3. World Health Organization, Memoranda, "A Revised System of Nomenclature for
   Influenza Viruses," *Bulletin, World Health Organization* 45 (1971), pp. 119–24. For
   detailed discussion, see also Walter R. Dowdle, Marion T. Coleman, and Michael B.
   Gregg, "Natural History of Type A in the United States," *Progress in Medical
   Virology* 17 (1974), pp. 91–135.
4. Martin M. Kaplan and Robert G. Webster, "The Epidemiology of Influenza,"
   Scientific American 237 (December 1977), pp. 88–106.
5. F. M. Burnet and Ellen Clark, *Influenza: A Survey of the Last 50 Years in the Light of
   Modern Work on the Virus of Epidemic Influenza* (London and Melbourne: Macmillan,
   1942).

6. William S. Jordan, Jr., "The Mechanism of Spread of Asian Influenza," *American Review of Respiratory Disease* 83 (1961), pp. 29–34.

7. E. H. Lennette, E. R. Rickard, G. K. Hirst, and F. L. Horsfall, Jr., "The Diverse Etiology of Epidemic Influenza," *Public Health Reports* 56 (1941), pp. 1777–88.

8. E. R. Rickard, Edwin H. Lenette, and Frank L. Horsfall, Jr., "A Comprehensive Study of Influenza in a Rural Community," *Public Health Reports* 55 (1940), pp. 2146–67.

9. Selwyn Collins, "Influenza and Pneumonia Excess Mortality at Specific Ages in the Epidemic of 1943–44, with Comparative Data for Preceding Epidemics," two parts, U.S. Public Health Service, *Public Health Reports* 60, no. 29 (July 20, 1945), pp. 821–35, and vol. 60, no. 30 (July 27, 1945), pp. 853–63.

10. Idem, "Age and Sex Incidence of Influenza in the Epidemic of 1943–44, with Comparative Data for Preceding Outbreaks," *Public Health Reports* 59, no. 46 (November 17, 1944), pp. 1483–1503.

11. U.S. Public Health Service, "Prevalence of Communicable Disease in the United States," *Public Health Report* 56, no. 7 (February 14, 1941), pp. 259–63.

12. Selwyn Collins, "Excess Deaths from Influenza and Pneumonia and from Important Chronic Disease During Epidemic Periods 1918–1951," Public Health Monograph no. 10 (Washington, D.C.: U.S. Department of Health, Education and Welfare, Public Health Service, 1951).

13. F. L. Horsfall, Jr., E. H. Lennette, E. R. Rickard, and G. K. Hirst, "Studies on the Efficacy of a Complex Vaccine Against Influenza A," *Public Health Reports* 56 (1941), pp. 1863–75.

14. Collins, "Influenza and Pneumonia Excess Mortality."

15. Gover, "Influenza and Pneumonia Mortality."

16. Collins, "Excess Deaths from Influenza."

17. U.S. Public Health Service, "Morbidity and Mortality from Specific Causes During 1943 and Recent Preceding Years," *Public Health Reports* 59 (1944), pp. 1047–65.

18. Collins, "Age and Sex Incidence of Influenza."

19. Ibid., "Influenza and Pneumonia Excess Mortality."

20. The Commission on Acute Respiratory Diseases, Fort Bragg, North Carolina, "The Periodicity of Influenza," *American Journal of Hygiene* 43 (1946), pp. 29–37.

21. The data for the following maps were extracted from vols. 58 (1943) and 59 (1944) of *Public Health Reports*.

22. Thomas Francis, Jr., Jonas E. Salk, and J. J. Quilligan, "Experience with Vaccination Against Influenza in the Spring of 1947," *American Journal of Hygiene* 37 (1947), pp. 1013–16.

23. Jonas E. Salk, Wilber J. Menke, Jr., and Thomas Francis, Jr., "A Clinical, Epidemiological and Immunological Evaluation of Vaccination Against Epidemic Influenza," *American Journal of Hygiene* 42 (1945), pp. 57–94.

24. A. P. Kendal et al., "Laboratory-Based Surveillance of Influenza Virus in the United States During the Winter of 1977–78, Part I: Periods of Prevalence of H1N1 and H3N2 Influenza A Strains, Their Relative Rates of Isolation in Different Age Groups and Detection of Antigenic Variants. Part II: Isolation of a Mixture of A/Victoria and A/USSR—Like Viruses from a Single Person During an Epidemic in Wyoming, USA, January 1978," *American Journal of Epidemiology* 110, no. 4 (1979), pp. 4349–67.

25. Gover, "Influenza and Pneumonia Mortality."

26. Allan Pred, "The Concentration of High Value-Added Manufacturing," *Economic Geography* 41 (1965), p. 111.

27. M. S. Pereira, "Global Surveillance of Influenza," *British Medical Bulletin* 35 (1979), pp. 9–14.

5
New Events and Old Assumptions: The 1950s

The worldwide pandemic of Asian strain influenza during 1957 was the most dramatic epidemiology phenomenon since the pandemics of influenza in 1918 and in 1889–1890. The accuracy of the predictions, the duration of the advanced warnings and the scope of the effort to control it in this country are unique in the history of organized medicine and public health.[1]

In these words, Alexander Langmuir explained the magnitude of the Asian (H2N2) influenza pandemic of 1957 and what was done about it in the United States. Actually, three major epidemics of influenza occurred in the 1950s. The first two, in 1951 and 1953, were caused by the 1947 (H1N1) strain, and the third was part of the Asian influenza pandemic of 1957. The latter event was *new* because a different strain of influenza was introduced into the population. Existing paradigms about geographical origins of pandemics were maintained, since the assumption that new strains of influenza spread from China seemed to be reinforced.

Other expected differences are also apparent when comparing spatiotemporal distributions of the 1950s epidemics. While the 1951 influenza outbreak was considered epidemic by some,[2] excessive mortality rates were more localized than the geographically wide-spread epidemic of 1953. The diffusion patterns of influenza caused by the genetically shifted 1957 virus were, in turn, considerably different from those of 1953, which were probably the result of a "drifting" virus. The 1957 pandemic was a dramatic epidemiological event; hence, most of this chapter is devoted to the geography of Asian (H2N2) influenza. Still, a greater understanding of the impact of viral shift on diffusion patterns is gained by first examining influenza geography in the United States immediately prior to the introduction of the new strain.

The Early 1950s: Some Familiar Tendencies

As the 1947 (H1N1) viral type of influenza, then known alternately as A-prime and A1, continued to prevail during the early 1950s, laboratory and epidemiological findings also accumulated. Many aspects of the periodicity of influenza and the appearance of new strains of the disease were clarified in light of the possible genetic shift that had taken place in the late 1940s. Two important aspects of the worldwide appearance of H1N1 that were noted by Francis in 1953 were just as important twenty-five years later (see Chapter 7).[3] The first observation was that H1N1 appeared in Australia in 1946 (with possible earlier origins in the Orient), spread to the United States in 1947, and reached Europe by 1948. This account thus supports the xenogenic paradigm that tends to permeate the epidemiological literature even as late as the 1950s. Second, Francis argued in favor of close genetic ties between the H1N1 strain and Hsw1N1 (swine) influenza that may have contributed to the 1918–19 pandemic. This likely association was reaffirmed in 1980.

Additional new notions about influenza spread and periodicity were put forth during the early 1950s as various analyses were consolidated. Andrewes believed that it was likely that "underground" diffusion of influenza can occur during nonepidemic periods. On the basis of studies that showed antibodies to strains of influenza without epidemic conditions, it was postulated that the disease may spread at times only among a small number of susceptible individuals in some form of seeding. The possibility of some individuals acting as "superspreaders" or avirulent—that is, symptomless or "silent"—carriers was also put forth. Many medical researchers were still dubious about the need for a permanent influenza surveillance network. Arguing in favor of the World Health Organization network established as a result of the 1946 epidemic, Andrewes stated:

> The virus must be able to loose itself from its restraint and get going in epidemic form with difficulty and infrequently. Thus it failed to do so anywhere for the great part of the 1954–55 winter. But when it does loose itself, it ravages a large part of the world within a few months. Let's accept what we see at its face value and admit that the country to country spread is a genuine phenomenon. It insures that over a large part of the globe the population is well seeded with one or a very limited number of antigenic types of viruses. In due course the outbreaks subside and virus persists, if at all, in a relatively avirulent state.[4]

Hence, the probability that the pending pandemic of 1957 would happen sometime in the future was a real consideration for influenza researchers. Before analyzing the spatial diffusion of the 1957 pandemic, it is useful for comparative purposes to examine geographical patterns of a prevailing strain with reference to what was actually known about influenza viruses at that time.

A comparison of the influenza outbreaks of 1951 and 1953 indicates that some spatiotemporal trends were similar to those of both the early 1940s and the late 1960s (see Chapter 6). Epidemic conditions were nearly met during February and March of 1951 as influenza flared up first along the Eastern Seaboard and then the West Coast.[5] The disease waned in the spring, however, which indicates the continuing circulation of a prevailing viral strain. Indeed, laboratory reports confirmed the continuing presence of Influenza A-prime (H1N1).[6]

The 1953 epidemic was more severe and widespread than the 1951 outbreak. The comparative mortality trends in Figure 5.1 show the magnitude of the 1953 epidemic in relation to the three preceding years.[7] An epidemic alert was issued by the United States Public Health Service early in January, when the influenza death rate exceeded the norm.[8] By mid-month, reports from military installations also indicated higher-than-normal morbidity.[9] Influenza-mortality rates remained higher than average for the civilian population throughout January and early February.[10] Also, reports of increasing

Deaths from Influenza and Pneumonia

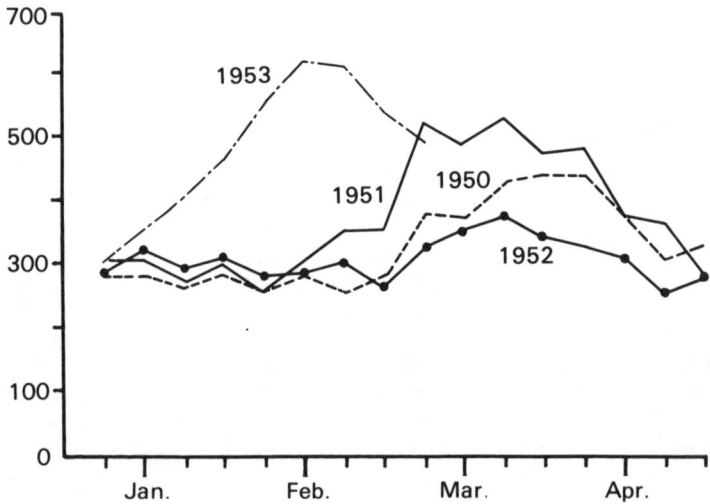

Figure 5.1. Springtime influenza mortality during the early 1950s. For several decades, the slightly drifted 1947 form of H1N1 was referred to as the "1951 strain." The trends shown here are largely due to that strain.

prevalence of influenza and other respiratory infections came from Europe, Africa, and the Far East. Viruses isolated in the United States and various parts of the world continued to be similar to those first identified in the late 1940s. In the United States mortality remained high during February, but the epidemic lost velocity near the end of the month as deaths decreased.[11]

A general impression of the spatial extent of the 1953 epidemic can also be obtained from Public Health Service documents.[12] The maps in Figures 5.2 and 5.3 show how localized outbreaks in Colorado, Oklahoma, Missouri, and North Carolina in December 1952 led to the subsequent diffusion of the disease through most of the central United States and some parts of the East by mid-January 1953. Also, by mid-January influenza had spread to most of the Southeast and to some western states. When the disease waned in February, declines in mortality reports were first noted within central parts of the country. Elevated influenza mortality continued into March along the fringes of the epidemic core area.

It is difficult to determine exactly why influenza did not spread outward from the central core area to coastal regions during the spring of 1953, but there are two possible explanations. The first and most logical is that the incidence of influenza decreased in the spring along with increasing temperatures. The second explanation is that since the 1951 flare-up was concentrated more heavily on the East and West coasts, there were fewer susceptible individuals in those regions. Still, temporal trends shown in Figure 5.1 suggest the possibility of genetic drift of the influenza virus.

Endemic Conditions in the Mid-1950s

Three years after the 1953 epidemic, there was another noticeable period of increased influenza activity. While not considered an epidemic period, the entire year before the emergence of the shifted virus that caused the 1957 pandemic was characterized by different forms of abnormal influenza reporting. More viral drift may have occurred, but isolates from several parts of the world indicated the continued presence of the 1947 (H1N1) type. This phenomenon— the increased reporting of a prevailing strain just prior to the clear identification of a new (or recycled) influenza virus—has turned out to be fairly common in recent decades. For example, the same thing seems to have happened during the 1967–68 and 1975–76 seasons, and perhaps also in the winter of 1946–47.

The first domestic indications of elevated levels of influenza activity were in the form of higher-than-average mortality from the disease in

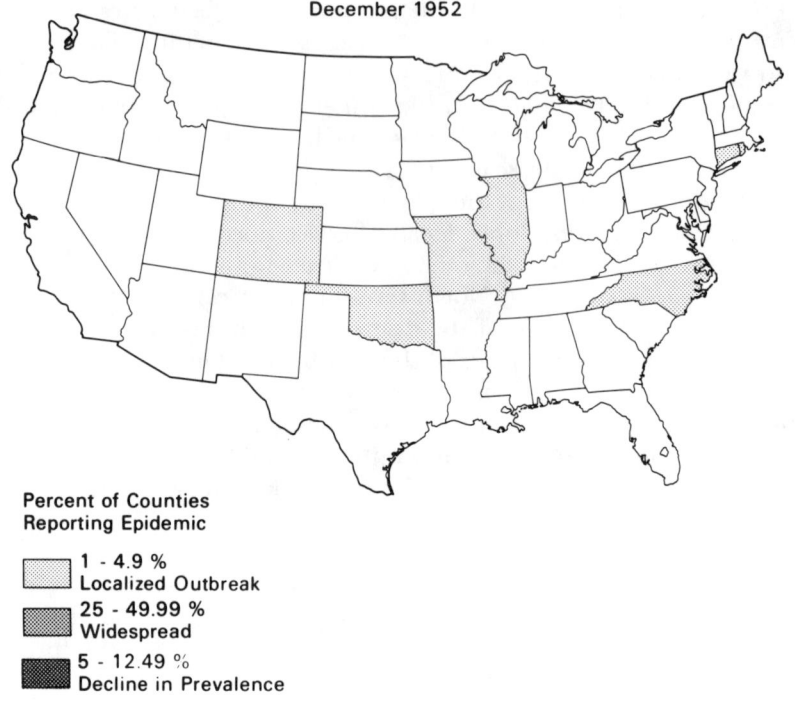

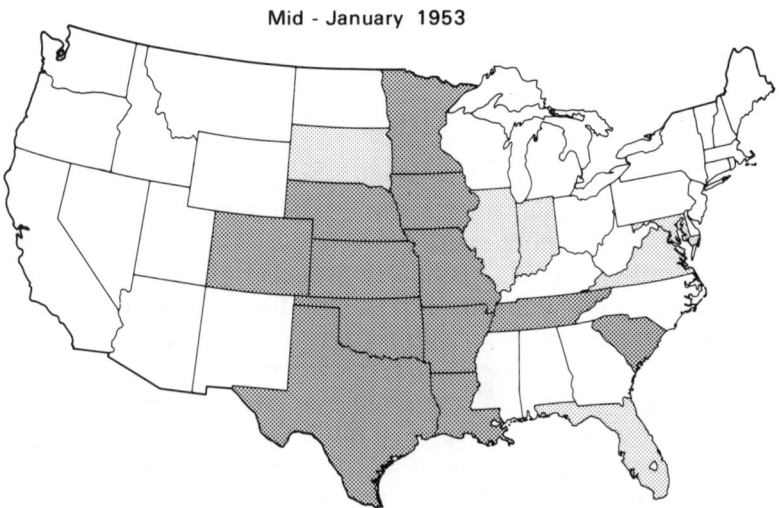

Figure 5.2. Morbidity reporting during the winter of 1952–53 indicated that the epidemic was most widespread in the central parts of the United States.

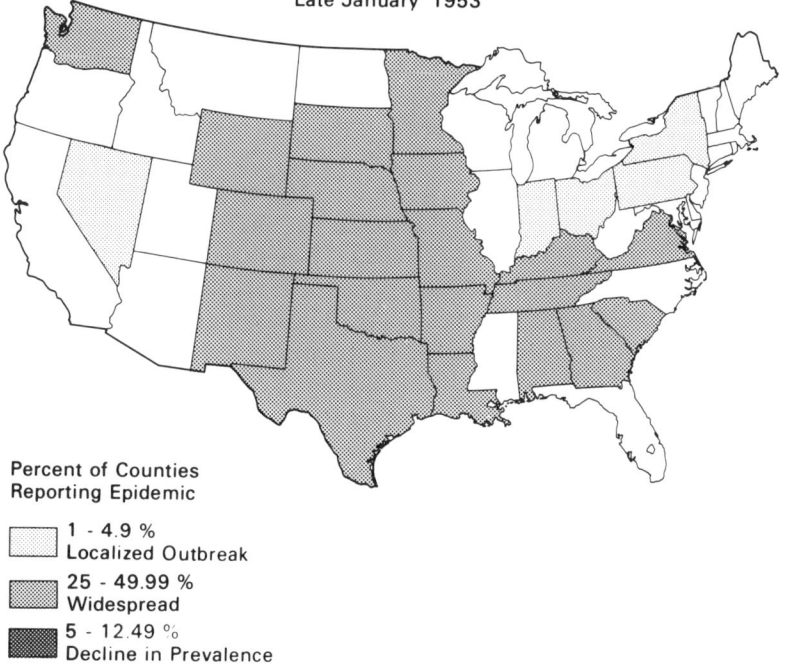

Late January 1953

Percent of Counties
Reporting Epidemic

1 - 4.9 %
Localized Outbreak

25 - 49.99 %
Widespread

5 - 12.49 %
Decline in Prevalence

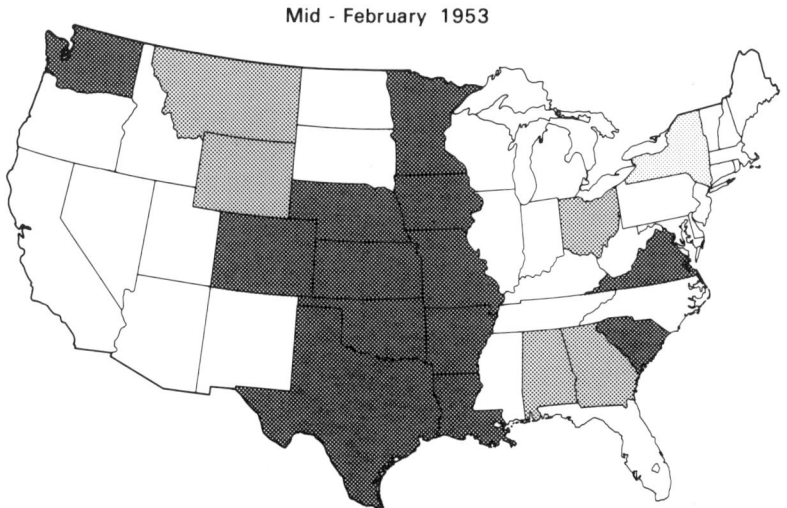

Mid - February 1953

Figure 5.3. By late winter the epidemic had spread somewhat from its central core area, but not all parts of the country were equally affected.

California, Ohio, and Colorado during March 1956.[13] Once again, forms of the 1947 (H1N1) virus were isolated in those locations. In March 1956 outbreaks of influenza also occurred in Austria, Italy, Switzerland, Spain, the United Kingdom, Yugoslavia, and Japan. However, no large-scale epidemic or extremely high mortality rates had been observed. Viral strains isolated in Europe continued to be similar to the "A-prime" types. By mid-March 1956 there were reports of mild outbreaks of influenza at scattered American universities, and there was a mild epidemic in Jamaica.[14] By late March influenza was considered epidemic among members of the United States armed forces in Britain, and civilian influenza-mortality rates were higher than normal for that time of the year.[15] In April influenza waned in both the Southern and Northern hemispheres.

The summer of 1956 was not characterized by unusual influenza activity within the Northern Hemisphere, but a mild epidemic of the disease began in Japan in October.[16] The outbreak apparently began on Shikoku Island and spread to the other major Japanese islands in November and December. The epidemic was relatively mild and occurred mostly within the school-age population. Both influenza A and B were isolated in Tokyo.[17] Such a dual pattern of viral activity had also characterized the 1947–48 epidemic, and this phenomenon occurred during the 1977–78 epidemic (see Chapter 7). Many United States armed forces personnel stationed in Japan also apparently contracted this form of influenza, and in January 1957 a mild outbreak was reported at a Colorado Air Force base.[18] Two strains of A-prime were isolated in Colorado, and the World Health Organization stated that isolates from the Japanese epidemic were serologically similar to the virus identified in the Netherlands in 1956.[19]

Reports of increased prevalence of influenza among both military and civilian populations continued during the spring of 1957. They included outbreaks below the epidemic threshold among United States personnel stationed in Korea as well as Japan.[20] Meiklejohn found that the A-prime virus isolated at an Air Force base in Colorado was similar to a type identified in Ann Arbor, Michigan, in 1956.[21] Additional reports of a mild influenzalike illness were recorded for Tennessee and South Carolina (both civilian and military), and an outbreak of respiratory infection took place in mid-February in the Pacific Northwest.[22] In February 1957 the Naval Research Unit at Great Lakes, Illinois, sent a preliminary report of a possible new influenza strain to the Public Health Service.[23] An outbreak of influenza occurred there in December 1956 and January 1957. When isolates were compared with other A-prime strains, they showed a marked difference in genetic composition. The Navy also reported the isolation of strains of A-prime at installations in Memphis, Tennessee, and Norfolk, Virginia. About the same time, Davenport identified five different strains of influenza in Michigan.[24]

Reports of influenzalike respiratory outbreaks and the isolation of A-prime viruses continued into March 1957. Even though no drastically different virus had yet been specifically identified, several types of the H1N1 group were circulating in widespread locations. In addition to the places already mentioned, flare-ups were reported in Arkansas, Iowa, and Pennsylvania.[25] In all of those episodes, sets of contiguous counties were involved. Outbreaks were also reported in the United Kingdom, Poland, and Scandinavia. Laboratory tests from an outbreak in southern Minnesota confirmed the presence of both A-prime and, interestingly, the PR8 laboratory virus. Most of the European viruses identified were similar to the Netherlands 1956 strain.

The reports of April 1957 were similar to those of previous months. The New York State Department of Health reported more isolations of A-prime, as did the Rhode Island Department of Health.[26] At the International Influenza Center of the Americas in Montgomery, Alabama, an analysis of eighteen isolates showed antigenic overlap between 1956 and 1957 sets of viruses then identified.[27] Similar findings were announced in Ohio and New Mexico.[28] During the spring of 1957, all indications were that known prevailing strains of influenza continued to circulate, although at a higher-than-normal rate. The increase of influenza activity and the extent of probable drift of the A virus suggested a high level of immunity. In addition, multiple minor cocirculating variants seemed to be, in restrospect, further conditions suitable for a shift and then a pandemic.

The Origin and Diffusion of the 1957 H2N2 Pandemic

In early May 1957 an epidemic of a disease presumed to be influenza was reported in Hong Kong; the type of virus probably responsible for the episode had yet to be determined. After several months of geographical backtracking, most epidemiologists agreed that a strain of shifted influenza virus had surfaced in China early in 1957.[29] Meanwhile, the disease was spreading outward from Southeast Asia.[30]

WORLDWIDE DIFFUSION PATHWAYS

The new strain of influenza, initially referred to as "Asian," had rapidly spread from Hong Kong to Japan, the Philippines, Malaya, and Indonesia by the end of May. By June there were numerous reports of influenza among passengers and crews of ships that had departed from East Asian ports,[31] and Australian port cities had become places of entry into that country.[32]

During June the disease also spread through India and the Middle East, and port cities were some of the first places to be affected. Given the nature of international trade ties, it was not surprising that the new strain of influenza had surfaced in England, as well as both the East and West coasts of the United States, by mid-summer. During July and August the new strain subsequently spread through Africa and South America. Accounts of the diffusion of influenza within the Soviet Union vary. In spite of the proximity of Vladisvostok to other Asian ports, some reconstructions of the epidemic indicate that the disease was present in Moscow in May. However, upon return from a visit to Soviet virological laboratories in June 1957, Albert Sabin reported that a virus not specifically identified had been spreading from the Far East along transportation lines.[33] World Health Organization information agreed with that conclusion.

DIFFUSION PATTERNS IN THE UNITED STATES

According to most accounts, the new strain of influenza entered the United States in June 1957.[34] Outbreaks of influenzalike illness had been reported at the Naval Training Station in San Diego, California, as well as aboard a naval vessel that had deployed from Newport, Rhode Island, to Norfolk, Virginia.[35] Laboratory tests also confirmed "Asian" influenza at military installations in Hawaii. By early July serologic tests indicated the presence of the H2N2 virus in a variety of locations.[36] The virus continued to surface in both military and civilian populations in California, Virginia, and Ohio; cases were also confirmed in Iowa.[37] In addition, there was speculation that the "new" strain may have been an older, recycled virus. For example, laboratory tests of elderly persons in several widespread locations showed antibodies against the Asian strain.[38] Similar tests in other locations indicated a strong chance that the current virus was closely related to the agent that caused the 1889–92 pandemic. Regardless of the history of the viral type, the possibility of death from influenza and pneumonia was a real threat to such high-risk groups as the elderly, and the Public Health Service had issued an alert by the summer of 1957.[39]

While later studies of the geographical spread of the disease indicated that it generally seems to have spread mostly from the West Coast eastward, with the same kinds of inland movements from the East Coast and the Gulf Coast, preliminary reports during the summer of 1957 were somewhat confusing. After outbreaks in California, there was some evidence that influenza then spread to Utah and

California. An outbreak in Iowa was then attributed to a group of students traveling from California to New York City.[40] However, there were also reports of epicenter formation at about the same time within the Chicago area, Kentucky, Ohio, New Mexico, Connecticut, and Maryland.[41] By August reports were coming in from Louisiana, Colorado, South Carolina, and Pennsylvania.[42]

Various incidents of the diffusion of influenza within small groups are also recorded. For example, Morris Greenburg of the New York City Department of Health reported to the Public Health Service an outbreak of influenza within a group of foreign-exchange students.[43] The students had traveled from Istanbul via Belgrade and Rotterdam. They were not permitted to board a ship bound for the United States. Instead, they were flown to New York City and nine were ill when they arrived. The New York State Department of Health also concluded that influenza had been carried by military transport from Germany, and in Minnesota an outbreak was blamed on a group of Bahamian migrant corn-pickers.[44] The disease was also found among migrant workers in Massachusetts, and in New Jersey there was an outbreak in September within a fishing fleet. In both the Panama Canal Zone and Puerto Rico, the incidence of influenza was high, thus adding to an argument espoused by some that the disease had also spread northward from Latin America.

While morbidity reports continued to increase, mortality indicators did not suggest a pandemic, no doubt because of the time lag involved. There was also some reluctance on the part of the Public Health Service to admit domestic pandemic conditions during August 1957. For example, a statement from the August 23, 1957, *Morbidity and Mortality Weekly Report* read: "Up to the present time, mortality data from 114 cities in the United States show no evidence of an increase which might be attributed to influenza."[45] Within a week, reports of influenzalike illness were pouring into the Public Health Service. The explosive nature of the H2N2 pandemic was obvious, and mortality counts had begun to increase by late September. Much of the summertime morbidity had been in school-age children, and when schools opened in the autumn, absenteeism because of influenza was high. This phenomenon is important: It could easily have been what was identified in the early 1980s as a form of herald wave. Morbidity from the disease seemed to have peaked by mid—October, but mortality was widespread. Some parts of the United States lagged behind others. These somewhat isolated locations included the Northern Plains areas, interior Texas, and parts of Appalachia.[46] By mid-November it was clear that as morbidity within the more youthful population declined, mortality among the elderly began to increase.

As information about the spread of the disease continued to

accumulate, it became increasingly clear that it had entered the country in widespread locations during the summer of 1957. A British precedent may also have been set, thus further explaining early outbreaks in New England. A comparison, released by the Public Health Service in November, suggested that H2N2 mortality peaked first during the autumn of 1957 in England and Wales and then in the United States (see Fig. 5.4).[47] Also, by August 1957 key counties had been selected for temporary morbidity reporting. County public health workers sent weekly summary data on influenza to a surveillance unit that had been established in Atlanta. Absenteeism was also monitored in selected industries. For example, the American Telephone and Telegraph Company, with its Bell system, cooperated in supplying daily absenteeism data from about 36 major United States cities to the Public Health Service. The National Healthy Survey, established in 1957, also estimated illness based on interviews of 700 households.

Using such data sources, Trotter and his associates surmised that summer outbreaks in various parts of the country served as multiple epicenters for the further diffusion of the disease.[48] They also indi-

Influenza Deaths

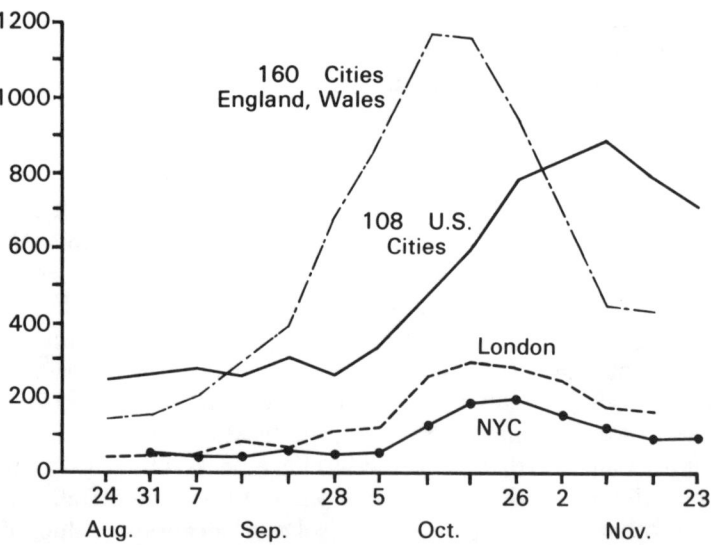

Figure 5.4. Influenza deaths during the H2N2 pandemic of 1957. Note that both England and Wales (and London) were affected, respectively, prior to the sample of U.S. cities and New York City.

cated general trends from July through October of massive diffusion from west to east and from the Gulf areas inland. Information on earliest outbreaks suggested epicenters forming in California, Montana, Arizona, and Florida. By September, Louisiana was one of the first states with at least half of its counties reporting substantial influenza morbidity. During the summer and fall of 1957 the Public Health Service also produced some maps in an attempt to follow the progression of the disease.[49] Adaptations of related Public Health Service maps in Figures 5.4, 5.5, and 5.6 show the distribution of what the Public Health Service identified as confirmed outbreaks, sporadic cases, and suspect outbreaks for civilian and military personnel for the time period July 29 to August 29, 1957.

It should be noted that by late July 1957 more than a dozen such centers were identified in California. By early August 1957, confirmed cases and/or outbreaks extended into Washington, Texas, Kentucky, Ohio, and Pennsylvania. By late August the disease appeared to be widespread throughout the West Coast, the Gulf Coast (including Florida), and many major cities in the Manufacturing Belt. Beginning in late September, the Public Health Service cartographic accounting system was changed from indicating outbreaks with dot patterns to maps showing which counties had actually reported influenza morbidity.[50] Figures 5.8 to 5.11 show the percentages of counties that had reported clear evidence of the epidemic. For example, the September 30, 1957, map shows heavier concentrations in some of the major epicenters already mentioned. By September the disease had become firmly established in the industrialized Northeast. Also, influenza had spread inland from most coastal areas. By mid-October 1957, in spite of the heavy concentrations of morbidity in the West, New York and Maine were the first to report more than 75 percent of their counties under epidemic conditions. By early November the states added to that list included Oregon, Alabama, New Jersey, Connecticut, Massachusetts, and Rhode Island. The epidemic continued to spread, and heavy concentrations emerged in Maryland, Ohio, Kentucky, West Virginia, and a general area along the western flank of the Appalachians.

Unlike some other phenomena associated with general diffusion analyses, this epidemic also did not spread in a hierarchical manner with respect to city size. Furthermore, there was no general outward diffusion from the more urbanized, industrialized parts of the country to other areas. Instead, the diffusion seemed to correspond to the sequential multiple-epicenter-formation pattern identified in Chapter 2.

Eventually, the epidemic led to numerous medical studies in specific locations. For example, Dunn and co-workers carried on exten-

Influenza - Far Eastern Strain - Confirmed and Suspect Cases, July 29, 1957

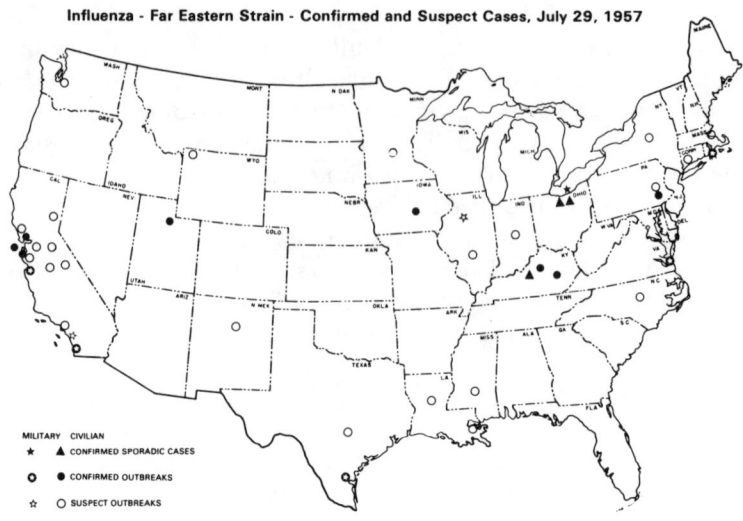

Influenza - Far Eastern Strain - Confirmed and Suspect Cases, August 5, 1957

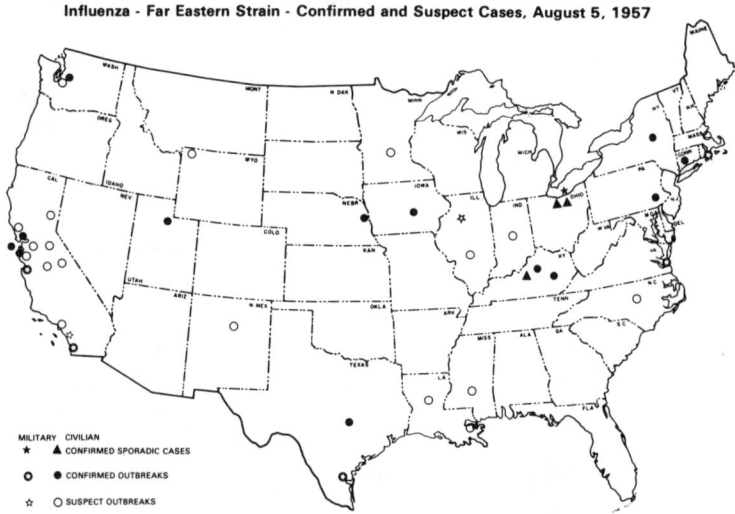

Figure 5.5. Morbidity reports, summer of 1957. The arrival of a new strain of influenza had been announced, and public health authorities were on the lookout for outbreaks and "sporadic" cases. The earliest epicenters seemed to form in California.

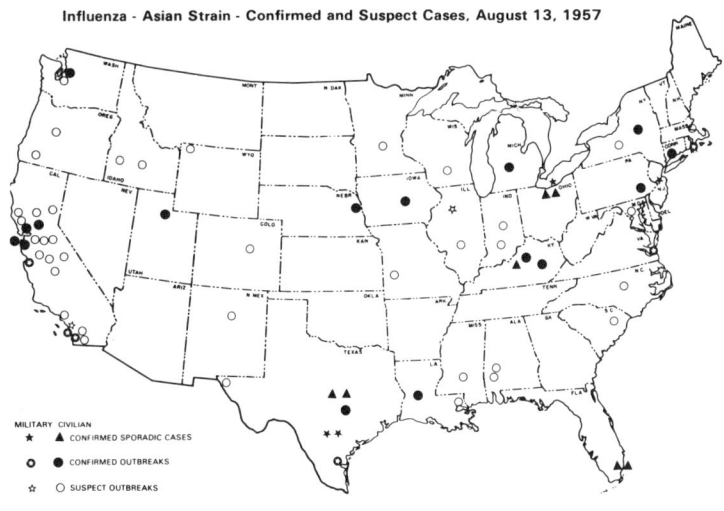

Influenza - Asian Strain - Confirmed and Suspect Cases, August 13, 1957

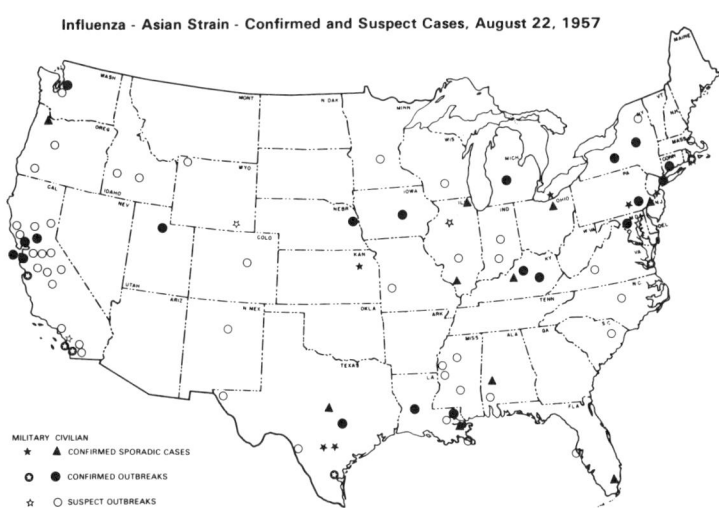

Influenza - Asian Strain - Confirmed and Suspect Cases, August 22, 1957

Figure 5.6. Continued influenza morbidity reporting during August 1957.

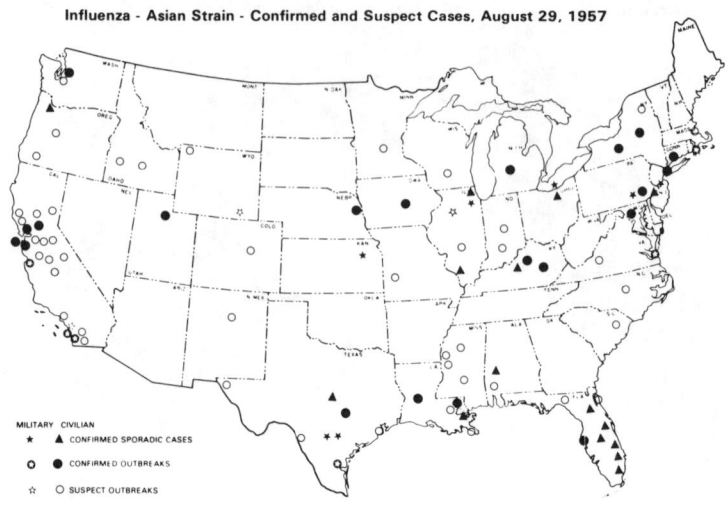

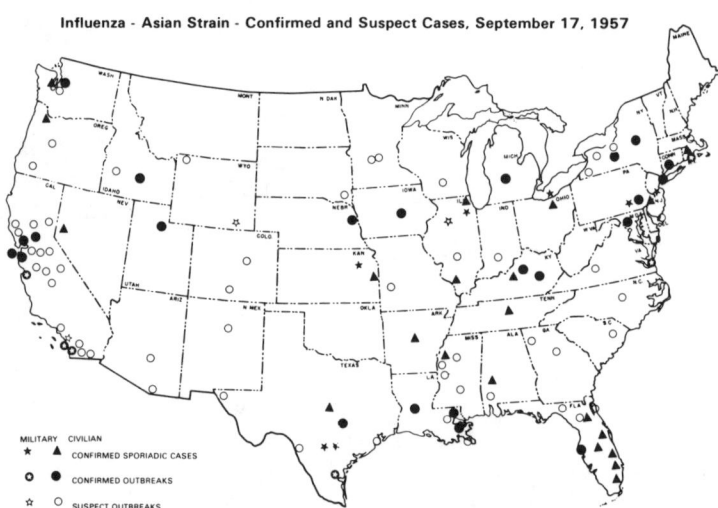

Figure 5.7. Epicenters had formed in several parts of the country by September 1957, according to morbidity reports.

sive epidemiological studies in the area of Louisiana where the disease was widespread.[51] Jordan and his colleagues developed similar studies in Cleveland, Ohio, and found that the virus was isolated in 41 percent of the families they studied.[52] Davenport and Hennessy, in an analysis of the epidemiology of Asian influenza, found that the typical mortality curve with high death rates among the very young and very old could be found in both Santiago, Chile, and Manila.[53] The age-mortality curve they identified was similar to that found in analyses of the 1928–29 influenza epidemic (see Chapter 3). However, evidence suggests that the earlier epidemic was not caused by the H2N2 virus.

In one of the most noteworthy studies of the 1957 epidemic, Langmuir showed how the overall mortality curve (as indicated by "excess" influenza and pneumonia deaths) peaked in November within the United States.[54] The excess mortality reports followed by several weeks the survelliance reports of higher morbidity during October. In one of the only known studies of that epidemic by geographers, Hunter and Young showed how influenza in England and Wales essentially followed the same kind of autumn peak on the first wave.[55] In addition, they identified mutliple epicenters that had formed in various parts of England and Wales, resulting in both major and minor diffusion foci. In fact, their study was also unique because general spatial-analytic techniques were used to test diffusion patterns against population potential.

SOME TEMPORAL SIMILARITIES WITH PAST PANDEMICS

Under influenza pandemic conditions, multiple temporal waves of mortality are common. During the late autumn of 1957, the epidemic within the United States appeared to dissipate. The lull was followed by yet another peak, or "wave," in early 1958 (Fig. 5.12).[56] Warmer temperatures during the spring and summer of 1958 contributed to declining influenza-pneumonia deaths. However, the winter of 1958–59 was also one of unusually high mortality. The virus then continued to circulate for the next decade. Such a temporal pattern seems to have been characteristic of the pandemics of 1889–92 and 1918–20.

Influenza Control: A Public or Private Matter?

As a result of the pandemic, major arguments had emerged about methods of influenza vaccine distribution. The central issue was whether the United States should rely exclusively on the private sector for inoculations during such a crisis or seriously consider national inoculation programs. A retrospective argument in favor of

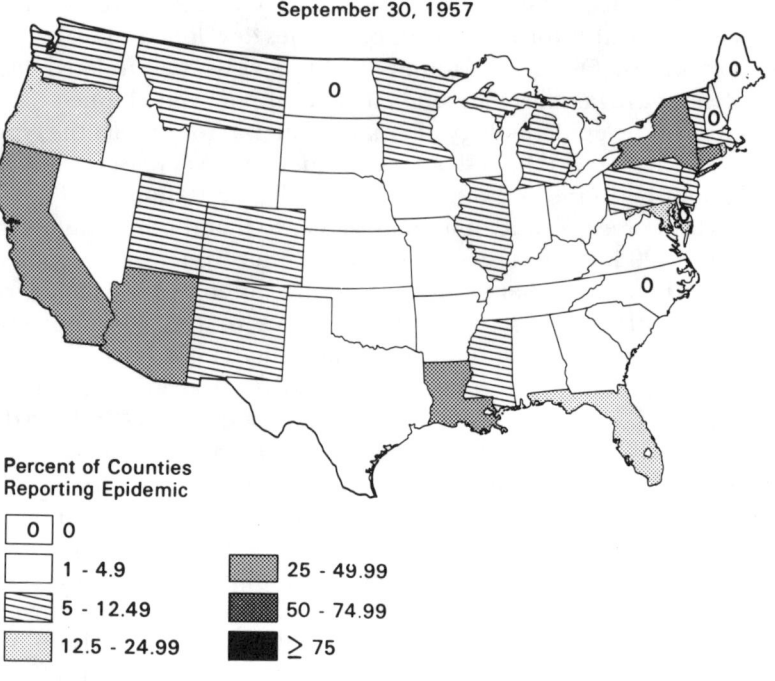

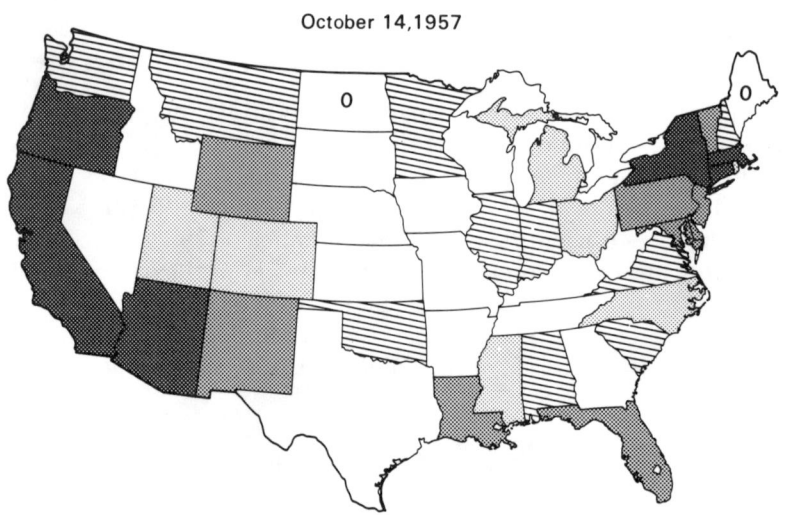

Figure 5.8. By September 1957, most counties in the United States had reported to the Public Health Service about epidemic conditions, defined simply as the presence or absence of sufficient morbidity. October epicenters on both the east and west coasts could be defined in this manner.

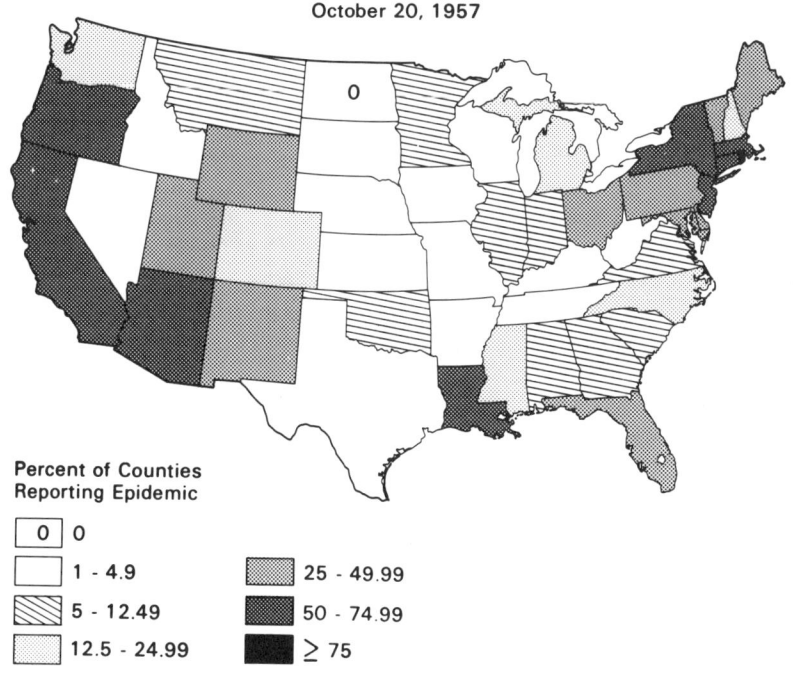

October 20, 1957

**Percent of Counties
Reporting Epidemic**

0	0
	1 - 4.9
	5 - 12.49
	12.5 - 24.99
	25 - 49.99
	50 - 74.99
	≥ 75

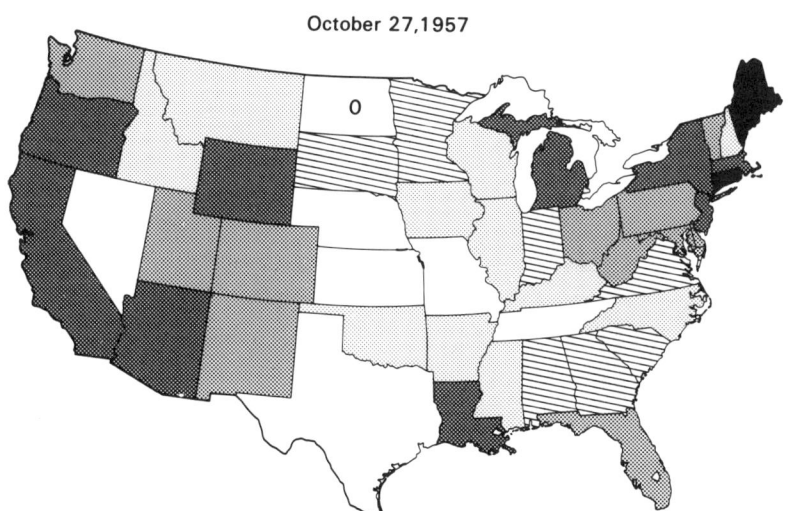

October 27, 1957

Figure 5.9. Continued use of morbidity reports in October 1957 showed how the epidemic seemed to spread from existing epicenters and also to form new ones in Louisiana and Michigan.

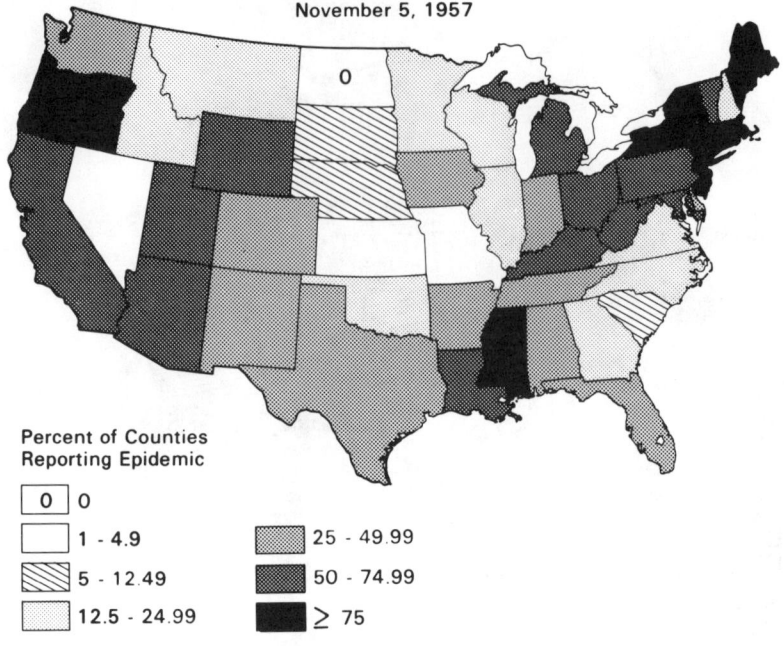

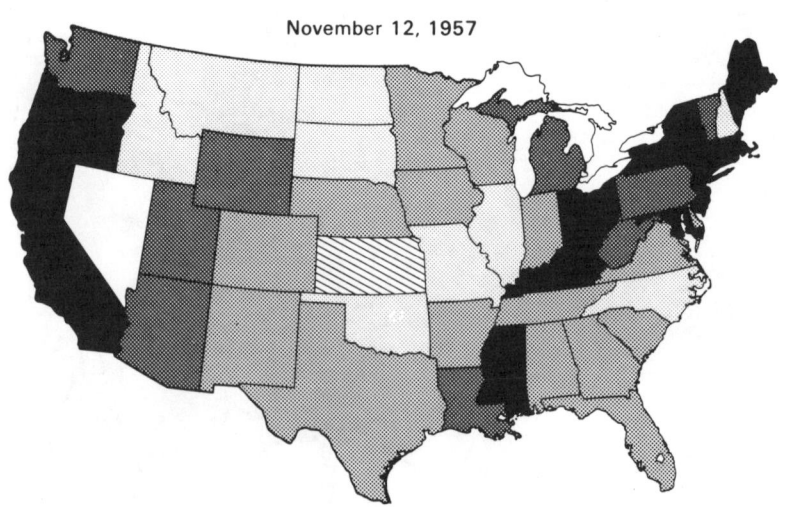

Figure 5.10. The continued spread of H2N2 morbidity during November 1957.

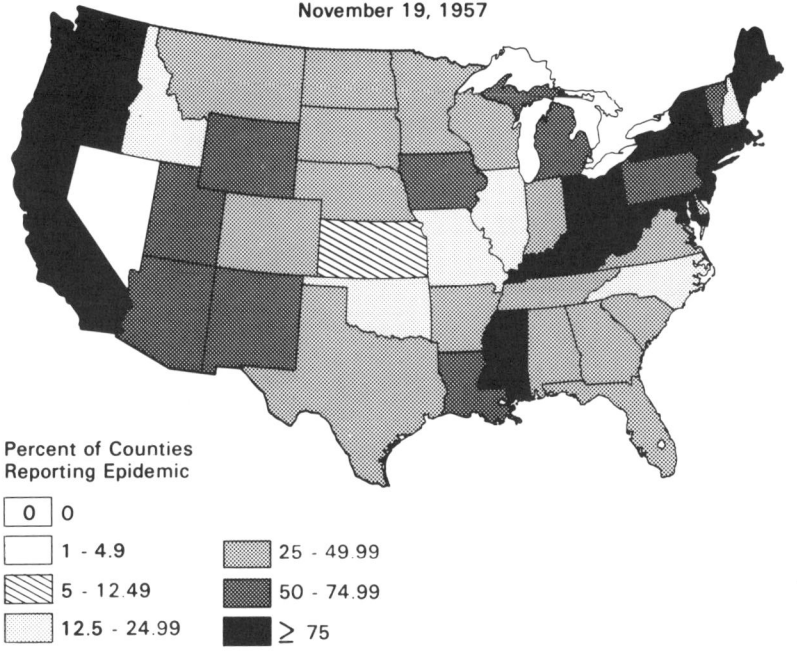

November 19, 1957

Percent of Counties
Reporting Epidemic

| 0 | 0 |

1 - 4.9

5 - 12.49

12.5 - 24.99

25 - 49.99

50 - 74.99

≥ 75

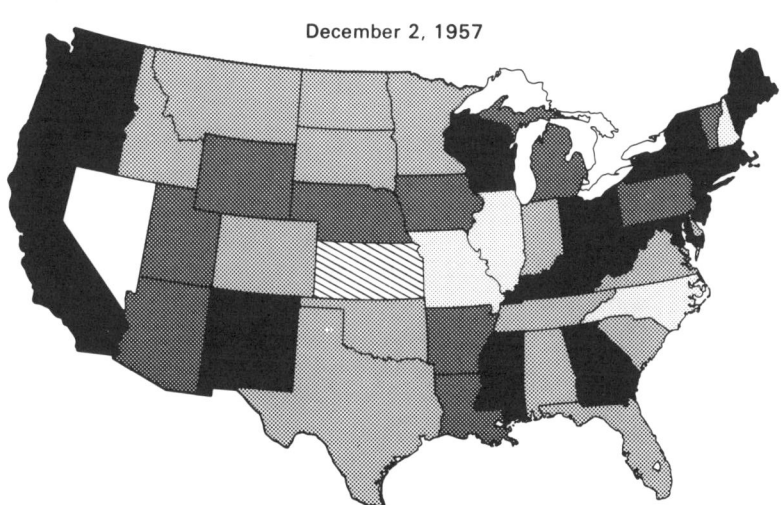

December 2, 1957

Figure 5.11. Continued morbidity reporting into early
December 1957.

UNITED STATES — 108 CITIES
Number of Deaths Associated
with Influenza-like Illness

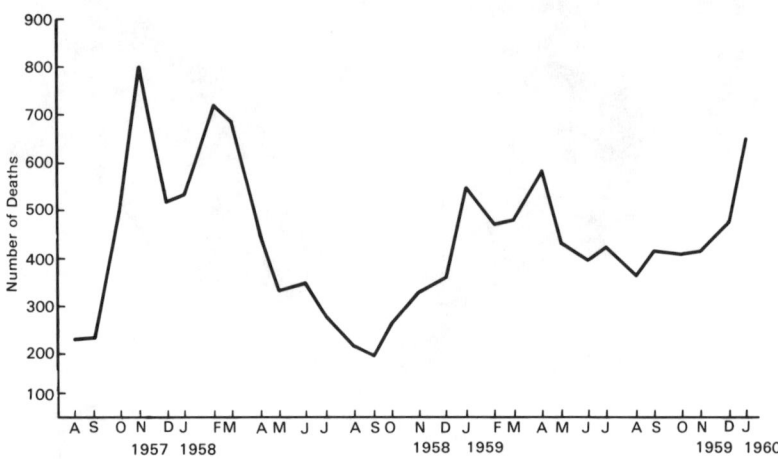

Figure 5.12. Retrospective analyses of influenza mortality during the 1957 pandemic indicated a series of subsequent waves of deaths lagging behind morbidity.

massive public inoculation programs is that as many as 80,000 people may have died prematurely because of the H2N2 influenza epidemic.[57] Clearly, inoculation programs serve several purposes: They prevent premature deaths among the elderly, curtail disease, and reduce school and work absenteeism. In fact, a procedure for a publicly supported inoculation program had been considered,[58] and there was ample lead time. While the "official" alert came from Leroy E. Burney, Surgeon General of the United States, in the September 1957 issue of *Public Health Reports,*[59] the Public Health Service had knowledge of the problem as early as the end of May. Preparations were made for the development and dissemination of a vaccine to combat H2N2. During the summer of 1957, a vaccination program had been planned. No major outbreaks were anticipated before the autumn of 1957, the normal beginning of most influenza epidemics, and vaccine manufacturers and policy makers alike were cautious about the specific type of vaccine to be developed.[60] Available information suggested that existing vaccines had little effect on the new virus. Several vaccines had to be studied to determine which one might be most effective. As early as June, a specific vaccine was adopted. But even by late June, the National Institutes of Health simply offered alternatives for action in the form of a "framework of alternatives." Many felt that the situation did not necessarily warrant the large-scale production and dissemination of vaccine by the United States government. The decision was made to allow the private sector to administer inoculations to the civilian populations on a voluntary basis.

There were many problems with the allocation and distribution of influenza vaccine. For example, according to Davis, the Public Health Service had sufficient warning of the 1957 epidemic to estimate its impact to some degree. However, there was a limited supply of vaccine. Davis also stated: "Unfortunately, the heavy civilian demand usually comes when cases begin to occur and are reported in official documents and in the press. As we know, vaccine must be administered about a month prior to the peak of an epidemic."[61] If a public program was to be adopted, the management of the distribution of vaccine during the H2N2 pandemic would have been the responsibility of the individual states and various public health officials and medical professionals. There was no overall coordination initiated at the national level. In defense of federal policy, Stewart explained that the Surgeon General appeared before the Senate Committee on Appropriations to testify about the need for funds.[62] As finally enacted, a bill provided about $800,000 in additional funds to deal with the epidemic. Of that amount, $225,000 was allocated for the production and distribution of diagnostic reactants. Another $385,000 was allocated for influenza surveillance and laboratory services, $80,000 for data collection and dissemination, and $110,000 for public health information and health education. Also, $275,000 was transferred to influenza-control activities from funds previously appropriated for communicable-disease control, and standby authority was granted to transfer as much as $2 million of emergency funds to the President. While this was a clear beginning, in many respects it can be viewed as too little too late in light of the more than $135 million required for the inoculation of 40 million persons during the 1976 program. It seems that the United States medical profession was not prepared to support a national inoculation program in 1957. In addition, there was sufficient government uncertainty and technical debate over the feasibility of mass inoculations to cloud the results of the policy decision to allocate funds for prevention.[63]

Notes

1. Alexander D. Langmuir, "Asian Influenza in the United States," *Annals of Internal Medicine* 49 (1958), p. 483–92.
2. C. H. Andrews, "Influenza: Theme and Variations," *California Medicine* 84 (1956), pp. 375–80.

3. Thomas Francis, Jr., "Influenza: The Newe Acquayantance," *Annals of Internal Medicine* 39 (1953), pp. 203–21.
4. Andrewes, "Influenza," p. 378.
5. Fred M. Davenport, Albert V. Hennessy, and Thomas Francis, Jr., "Epidemiologic and Immunologic Significance of Age Distribution of Antibody to Antigenic Variants of Influenza Virus," *Journal of Experimental Medicine* 98 (1953), pp. 641–56.
6. Thomas Francis, Jr., "The Current Status of the Control of Influenza," *Annals of Internal Medicine* 43 (1955), pp. 534–38.
7. U.S. Public Health Service, "Provisional Information on Selected Diseases in the United States for Week Ended March 7, 1953," *Morbidity and Mortality Weekly Report* (hereafter referred to as *MMWR*), Washington, D.C.: Federal Security Agency, National Office of Vital Statistics, March 13, 1953. By the mid-1950s the Federal Security Agency had become a part of the Department of Health, Education and Welfare.
8. *MMWR* 1 (January 8, 1953), pp. 1–3.
9. *MMWR* 2 (January 16, 1953), pp. 1–3.
10. *MMWR* 2 (February 13, 1953), pp. 1–3.
11. Selwyn D. Collins and Josephine L. Lehmann, "Influenza Epidemics During 1951–56 with a Review of Trends," *Public Health Reports* 72 (1957), pp. 771–80.
12. *MMWR* 2 (February 20, 1953), pp. 1–4.
13. *MMWR* 5 (March 2, 1956), p. 1.
14. *MMWR* 5 (March 23, 1956), p. 1.
15. *MMWR* 5 (April 6, 1956), p. 1.
16. *MMWR* 5 (December 28, 1956), p. 1.
17. *MMWR* 6 (January 18, 1957), p. 1.
18. *MMWR* 6 (Jaunary 25, 1957), p. 1.
19. *MMWR* 6 (April 12, 1957), p. 1.
20. *MMWR* 6 (February 1, 1957), p. 1.
21. *MMWR* 6 (February 8, 1957), p. 1.
22. *MMWR* 6 (February 15, 1957), p. 1.
23. *MMWR* 6 (Feburary 27, 1957), pp. 1–2.
24. Fred M. Davenport, "Influenza Viruses," in A. S. Evans, ed., *Viral Infections in Humans: Epidemiology and Control* (New York: Plenum Medical Book Co., 1977), pp. 273–91.
25. *MMWR* 6 (March 8, 1957), p. 1.
26. *MMWR* 6 (April 5, 1957), pp. 1–2.
27. *MMWR* 6 (April 19, 1957), pp. 1–2.
28. *MMWR* 6 (April 26, 1957), pp. 1–2.
29. Keith E. Jensen and Ralph B. Hogan, "Laboratory Diagnosis of Asian Influenza," *Public Health Reports* 73 (1958), pp. 140–44.
30. *MMWR* 6 (May 31, 1957), p. 1–2.
31. World Health Organizations, "The 1957 Influenza Epidemic," *W.H.O. Chronicle* 2 (1957), pp. 269–71.
32. Frederick L. Dunn, "Pandemic Influenza in 1957," *Journal of the American Medical Association* 166 (1958), pp. 1140–48.
33. *MMWR* 6 (June 28, 1957), pp. 1–2.
34. *MMWR* 6 (June 21, 1957), pp. 1–2.
35. U.S. Public Health Service, "Asian Strain of Influenza A," *Public Health Reports* 72 (1951), pp. 768–70.
36. H. M. Meyer, Jr., M. R. Hillman, M. L. Miesse, I. P. Crawford, and A. S. Bankhead, "New Antigenic Variant in Far East Influenza Epidemic, 1957," *Proceedings, Society for Experimental Biology and Medicine* 95 (1957), pp. 604–16.
37. Alexander D. Langmuir, "Epidemiology of Asian Influenza," *American Review of Respiratory Diseases* 83 (1961), pp. 2–9.
38. Suzanne K. R. Clarke, R. B. Heath, R. N. P. Sutton, and C. H. Stuart-Harris, "Serological Studies with Asian Strain of Influenza A," *Lancet* 1 (1958), pp. 814–18; and J. Mulder and N. Masurel, "Pre-Epidemic Antibody Against 1957 Strain of Asiatic Influenza," *Lancet* 1 (1958), pp. 810—14.

39. Leroy E. Burney, "Influenza Epidemic Alert," *Public Health Reports* 72 (1957), p. 767.
40. Langmuir, "Epidemiology of Asian Influenza," p. 4.
41. *MMWR* 6 (July 12, 1957), p. 2.
42. *MMWR* 6 (August 2, 1957), pp. 1–2.
43. *MMWR* 6 (August 23, 1957), p. 1.
44. *MMWR* 6 (September 20, 1957), pp. 1–2.
45. *MMWR* 6 (August 23, 1957), pp. 1–2.
46. *MMWR* 6 (October 4, 1957), pp. 1–2.
47. *MMWR* 6 (November 30, 1957), p. 2.
48. Yates Trotter, Jr., Frederick L. Dunn, Robert H. Drachman, Donald A. Henderson, Mario Pizzi, and Alexander Langmuir, "Asian Influenza in the United States, 1957–1958," *Amercian Journal of Hygiene* 70 (1959), pp. 34–50.
49. Alexander D. Langmuir, Mario Pizzi, William Y. Trotter, and Frederick Dunn, "Asian Influenza Surveillance," *Public Health Reports* 73 (1957), pp. 114–20.
50. Ibid.
51. Frederick L. Dunn, Donald E. Carey, Arthur Cohen, and Joseph D. Martin, "Epidemiological Studies of Asian Influenza in a Louisiana Parish," *American Journal of Hygiene* 70 (1959), pp. 351–71.
52. William S. Jordan, Jr., Floyd W. Denney, Jr., George F. Badger, Constance Curtiss, John H. Dingle, Robert Oseasohn, and David A. Stevens, "A Study of Illness in a Group of Cleveland Families," *American Journal of Hygiene* 68 (1958), pp. 190–211.
53. Fred M. Davenport and Albert V. Hennessy, "The Clinical Epidemiology of Asian Influenza," *Annals of Internal Medicine* 49 (1958), pp. 493–501.
54. Langmuir, "Epidemiology of Asian Influenza."
55. John M. Hunter and Jonathan C. Young, "Diffusion of Influenza in England and Wales," *Annals, Association of American Geographers* 61 (1971), pp. 637–53.
56. Carl C. Dauer, "Morbidity in the 1957–58 Influenza Epidemic," *Public Health Reports* 73 (1958), pp. 803–10.
57. Dorland J. Davis, "Problems of Allocation and Distribution of Influenza Vaccines," *American Review of Respiratory Disease* 83 (1961), pp. 168–70.
58. William H. Stewart, "Administration History of the Asian Influenza Program" *Public Health Reports* 73 (1958), pp. 101–13.
59. Burney, "Influenza Epidemic Alert."
60. Gordon Meiklejohn and Alton J. Morris, "Influenza Vaccination," *Annals of Internal Medicine* 49 (1958), pp. 529–35.
61. Davis, "Problems of Allocation and Distribution of Influenza Vaccines."
62. Stewart, "Administration History of the Asian Influenza Program."
63. For example, Kilbourne et al. reiterated many of the views that prevailed in the late 1950s in a workshop sponsored by the National Institutes of Health more than a decade after the H2N2 pandemic. See *Journal of Infectious Diseases* 129 (1974), pp. 750–71.

References

Commission on Influenza. "Vaccination Against Asian Influenza." *Journal of the American Medical Association* 165 (1957), pp. 2055–58.

Davenport, Fred M. "Recent Advances in Prevention of Influenza by Vaccination." *Modern Medicine* 26 (1958), pp. 115–22.

Dull, H. Bruce, et al. "Monovalent Asian Influenza Vaccine." *Journal of the American Medical Association* 172 (1960), pp. 1223–29.

Hilleman, Maurice R., et al. "Antibody Response in Volunteers to Asian Influenza Vaccine." *Journal of the American Medical Association,* 166 (1958), pp. 1134–40.

Jensen, Keith E., Allen F. Woodhour and Ann A. Bailey. "Immunization with Polyvalent Influenza Vaccines." *Journal of the American Medical Association* 172 (1960), pp. 1230–38.

Smadel, Joseph E. "Influenza Vaccine." *Public Health Reports* 73 (1958), pp. 129–32.

6

The Ascendancy of
"Hong Kong" Influenza

The Asian (H2N2) strain of influenza examined in Chapter 5 continued to be the most pronounced type A variant internationally for
more than a decade. Then, in a fashion similar to that suggested by
Kilbourne (Chapter 1), a new strain emerged to supplant H2N2.
While both the specific geographical origins and subsequent patterns
of spatial diffusion of the newer strain were somewhat less clear than
during some earlier twentieth-century episodes involving genetic
shift, a variant classified now as A(H3N2) and in 1968 as "Hong
Kong" surfaced, probably first in China. Most contemporary accounts
suggest that it spread during the summer of 1968 through Hong
Kong across the Pacific Ocean to the United States, southward to
Australasia, and westward across both land and sea to Western
Europe.

Patterns of spatial diffusion were also less dramatic than during the
early phases of the introduction of H2N2 a decade or so earlier, and
there was some confusion about the possible nature of the new strain.
Descriptions of what actually happened during the pandemic were
also clearly less dogmatic than earlier accounts of the spread of the
disease. As stated by Sir Christopher Andrewes:

> I have been increasingly puzzled by the accounts of different incidence
> of Hong Kong influenza in different countries. I venture to put
> forward an hypothesis invented on the spur of the moment—might
> there not be 2 variants of the virus circulating around the world,
> differing in virulence and power of spread?[1]

Somewhat after Andrewes's observation, it was confirmed through
laboratory testing that one major new strain had emerged. But two
patterns of influenza diffusion had actually taken place. The first and
by far most common consisted of unusually high influenza mortality
from an existing strain during the winter season immediately prior to
the introduction of a new strain in pandemic form. Of course, we

have no exact way of knowing that an unusual flare-up of a prevailing influenza strain one winter will actually result in the introduction of a new strain. What is rather remarkable instead is that this phenomenon seems to have taken place prior to the pandemics of 1918, 1947, 1957, and 1968. In addition, it took place during the winter influenza season of 1967–68 in several parts of the world at somewhat different times. In other words, there is the strong possibility that some parts of the world were still witnessing excessive mortality from an unexpected epidemic of H2N2 when others first felt the impact of the arrival of H3N2. The second feature that seems characteristic of the introduction of H3N2 is that, for reasons yet to be fully explained, this variant of influenza takes on a diffusion pattern that is usually characterized by an outward spread from multiple epicenters. While an initial reaction might be that this form of spatial diffusion is somehow linked to modern airline travel, examples of the same type of spread were documented long before the invention of the internal combustion engine (Chapter 2). Still, multiple-epicenter diffusion is also common once a strain of influenza becomes well established within a geographical area. In fact, such was the case with H2N2 soon after its initial introduction. An examination of that circumstance along with an explanation of advances in influenza surveillance during the early 1960s add to our cumulative knowledge of the geography of the disease.

Further Observation on the Cyclical Nature of Influenza

The long-term studies by Selwyn Collins mentioned earlier serve as an excellent historical record of past epidemics. With the continued reductions in overall influenza-mortality trends in the twentieth century, it became increasingly apparent to influenza epidemiologists that the major utility of the "Collins method" was indeed the development of retrospective accounts. By the 1950s the cyclical nature of influenza was clearly well known, but the magnitude of the H2N2 epidemic could not be predicted with existing methodologies. It was only near the end of the second wave of the H2N2 pandemic that biostatisticians seriously started to explore methods of "early warning," at least within the context of "an early quantitative measure of the severity of an influenza epidemic and its geographical localization."[2]

The major surveillance method put forth by Serfling in the late 1950s served as the primary indicator of the severity of influenza mortality for more than two decades. In his capacity as chief of statistics in the Epidemiology Branch of the then-fledgling Communicable Disease Center, Serfling developed the new technique as a result of surveillance failures during the H2N2 pandemic. His rationale included several shortcomings of earlier procedures:

1. Reporting of influenza through routine physician reports was inadequate.
2. Laboratory tests could yield only qualitative indications of prevalence.
3. Epidemic reports from various locations lacked uniform quantitative standards.
4. Industrial and school absenteeism data were not widely available, even during the height of the epidemic.
5. The U.S. National Health Survey provided only weekly estimates based on a limited sample.

Actually, Serfling posited a new way to measure what epidemiologists had sought for a long time: excess mortality. In its simplest definition, excess influenza mortality is defined as the measurable amount of mortality during any given period in excess of what would normally be expected. The key to understanding Serfling's method is the term *expected.*

According to Serfling, three things were required to determine "advance estimation of expected pneumonia-influenza mortality levels":[3] (1) the determination of a "secular" trend; (2) an estimation of seasonal variations; and (3) a distinction between major departures from expected oscillations and random variation. In other words, he used Fourier series to identify cycles of normal reporting to determine "expected" deaths during any given week. Irregularities over time were removed by using the mathematical function:

$$\hat{Y} = u + bt + \Sigma_{a_i} \cos \theta + \Sigma_{b_i} \sin \theta$$

where θ is a linear function of t.

For more than twenty years the method was used with CDC city reporting data measured in four-week periods. Conditions were considered epidemic if actual reporting exceeded "expected" trends by some specified amount, such as 1.64 standard deviation; adjustments were periodically made. This method seemed to work best when the numerical effects of epidemics were removed. Tables were constructed with rows consisting of thirteen four-week periods, and columns were made up of four-week averages for the thirteen time periods over several years.[4] Standard seasonal curves were then determined to remove unusual minor variations. This procedure was deemed appropriate for short-term measurement purposes, but it worked best, as with the Collins method, within a retrospective context.

For purposes of longer-term forecasting, a double-integration method was used: means from observed values were theoretically set to values of an appropriate sine function and integrated twice:

$$\hat{Y} - \overline{Y} = A \sin \left[\frac{2\pi(h - 1)}{N} + \Phi\right];$$

where A = amplitude
  N = the number of periods, such as 13
and Φ = the phase angle with h = 1, 2 . . . N

Following such logic:

$$A \int_{\frac{1}{2}}^{h+\frac{1}{2}} \sin \left[\frac{2\pi(h - 1)}{N} + \Phi\right] dh = -\frac{AN}{2\pi} \cos \left[\frac{2\pi(h - \frac{1}{2})}{N} + \Phi\right]$$

with substitution of the mean,

$$\frac{AN}{2\pi} \cos \left(\Phi - \frac{\pi}{N}\right)$$

Right-side integration over the range h = $\frac{1}{2}$ to h + $\frac{1}{2}$ gives

$$\frac{-AN^2}{4\pi^2} \sin \left(\frac{2\pi h}{N} + \Phi\right)$$

after the mean is subtracted,

$$\frac{AN^2}{4\pi^2} \sin \Phi$$

An equivalent set of numerical computations was completed on the left side of the equation

$$Y_h - \overline{Y} = A \sin \left(\frac{2\pi(h + 1)}{N} + \Phi\right)$$

Instead of integration, however, summation was used

$$\sum_{1}^{h} (Y_h - \overline{Y}) = \frac{1}{N}\left[N \sum_{1}^{h} Y_h - h \sum_{-1}^{N} Y_h\right]$$

with a mean value over the range h = 1 to h = n of

$$\frac{1}{N}\left[\sum_1^N \sum_1^h Y_h - \left(\frac{N+1}{2}\right)\sum_1^N Y_h\right]$$

The mean was then subtracted from each term and cumulated, giving

$$\frac{1}{N}\left[N\sum_1^h \sum_1^h Y_h - h\sum_1^N \sum_1^h Y_h + \frac{h(N-h)}{2}\sum_1^N Y_h\right]$$

with a mean value of

$$\frac{1}{N}\left[\sum_1^N \sum_1^h \sum_1^h Y_h - \left(\frac{N+1}{2}\right)\sum_1^N \sum_1^h Y_h + \left(\frac{N^2-1}{12}\right)\sum_1^N Y_h\right]$$

Column totals

$$T_1 = \sum_1^N Y_h,$$

$$T_2 = \sum_1^N \sum_1^h Y_h, \text{ and}$$

$$T_3 = \sum_1^N \sum_1^h \sum_1^h$$

were computed in a cumulative fashion and used to construct tables
that also included the following terms:

$$S_h = 2NH - h(2T_2) + h(N - h)T_1,$$

$$C = -T_1\left(\frac{N^2-1}{6}\right) + (N+1)T_2 - 2T_3,$$

$$\text{and } \hat{Y}_{h+1} = \frac{T_1}{N} - \frac{2\pi^2}{N^3}(sh + c)$$

Actually, the estimating equation used was:

$$\hat{Y}_{h+1} = \bar{Y} + A\sin\left(\frac{2\pi h}{N} + \Phi\right) = \bar{Y} - \frac{2\pi^2}{N^3}(S_h + c)$$

Tables of these terms were constructed using "national" reporting
data from 108 key surveillance cities. They were, in turn, recalibrated
after most seasons to account for new mean values. Theoretically, this

method was more sophisticated than earlier systems, but in practice it fell far short of expectations primarily because only national and broad regional totals were used in the estimation process. The curves shown in Figure 6.1 give some indication of the "expected" (solid line) national rates during the H2N2 epidemic and the upper limit, or epidemic threshold (dashed line), as applied during early usage of the method. The problem, however, was that by the time an epidemic was recognized for the sum of the 108 cities, it had long since reached epidemic proportions in lead cities. Still, it was the most sophisticated method used by the Public Health Service for more than two decades.

Influenza Surveillance in the Early 1960s

One of the first analyses of the diffusion of *endemic* H2N2 was accomplished by Eikhoff and Robinson in 1961.[5] In what has subsequently become known as the "third wave" of the 1957 pandemic, Eikhoff and Robinson found little of the massive frontal movement that had been identified earlier by Trotter et al.[6] During January and February of 1960, the United States was suddenly faced with another epidemic of influenza.[7] Not only did the newly established surveillance methodology fail to predict the epidemic, but epidemiologists also had no idea how it might spread geographically. If fact, Eikhoff and Robinson uncovered a pattern of diffusion outward from multiple epicenters that was eventually to become characteristic of subsequent influenza-diffusion patterns in the 1960s. While such patterning is often indicative of the balance between immune and susceptible populations, it also suggests that a strain of the disease is well established within a large geographical area. However, such geographical establishment of an influenza strain does not necessarily mean that the health-care system is responding to the problem.

In what was with little doubt one of the most carefully written and accurately documented explanations of the influenza problem in the early 1960s, Eikhoff teamed up with Sherman and Serfling to co-

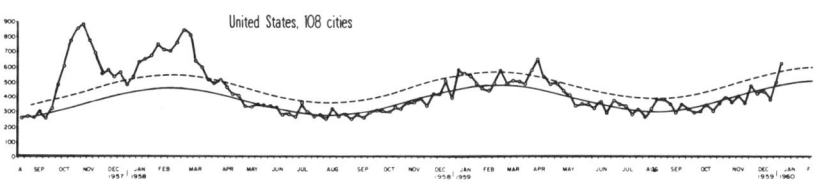

Figure 6.1. An application of Serfling's model to data from the 1957 pandemic.

author an article for the wide readership of the *Journal of the American Medical Association*.[8] They explained the newly defined concept of "excess mortality" in relation to recent epidemics by suggesting that as many as 86,000 high-risk individuals may have died prematurely from influenza. High-risk individuals include the elderly and others with lowered resistance. They also suggested that additional lives were probably lost through the indirect effects of viral infection, and many of the deaths primarily attributed to such health problems as cardiovascular-renal disease may have been triggered first by influenza. The contribution by Eikhoff et al. was strongly persuasive with respect to the need for routine and more widespread dissemination of the vaccine against H2N2. Their concluding comment was in fact a polite understatement aimed toward practicing physicians: "Immunologic protection through the routine use of influenza vaccine in such high-risk groups may be of great value in reducing the extent of influenza-associated excess mortality."[9]

Improvements were made in the surveillance network in the 1960s, and more attention was paid to the need for influenza inoculations. But the situation was complicated by yet another factor during a minor epidemic of the disease in January 1963: While there were some indications of an outbreak,[10] there was also sufficient genetic drift within the general H2N2 strain to cut down on the efficacy ratio of vaccines then in use. Again, geographical patterns of diffusion were not identified by epidemiologists, but it is of interest that California, with higher-than-average excess mortality during the 1960 epidemic, had fewer expected deaths during the 1963 episode. Polyvalent influenza vaccines were recommended, especially for high-risk groups.[11] It is also of interest that the Canadian experience with influenza epidemics was basically similar to that of the United States.[12] A major change was about to take place internationally, however, and it seems to have been heralded by extensive outbreaks of H2N2 during the winter of 1967–68 in both Britain and the United States.

Probable Origins and the Early Nature of H3N2 Diffusion

Most contemporary sources agree that the "Hong Kong" or H3N2 strain of influenza that emerged in the late 1960s probably had its origins somewhere on the Chinese mainland. In one of the more specific estimates, Hideo Fukumi narrowed the specific geographical locations to either Kweichow or Yunan.[13] While the new strain was first clearly identified in Hong Kong in mid-July 1968, it could easily have been spreading through various parts of China for several months. The new strain had some characteristics in common with

H2N2, but it immediately became clear that immunity to the earlier prevailing strain did not protect against the newly discovered strain. Other similarities and differences were immediately noticed with regard to spatiotemporal characteristics of the two strains. One important circumstance preceding the emergence of the new strain was an internationally widespread epidemic of H2N2 in the winter of 1967–68. Here is yet another example in the twentieth century of a substantial flare-up of an existing strain in the winter before a pandemic caused by a different virus. Patterns of spatial diffusion were fairly different between the two strains, however. Unlike the international spread of Asian influenza during the 1957 pandemic, H3N2 did not initially diffuse outward in massive frontal waves. Instead, it seems to have gone through a process of initial and slow multiple seeding and then diffused outward from several epicenters simultaneously. These phenomena had been recorded in different parts of the world at different times, and the latter aspect mentioned above was more than once referred to by epidemiologists as a sort of "smoldering" effect. Other accounts of the spread of the disease during the earliest phases of diffusion are somewhat curious because some influenza researchers contended that the pandemic was much worse in the United States than other parts of the world.[14] Subsequent evaluations of the intensity of the pandemic showed that in some instances the full impact of the arrival of H3N2 was simply stalled only for a year or so.

Diffusion of H3N2 from Hong Kong to other parts of the world is fairly well documented. But even though surveillance increased during the decades following major influenza epidemics, the World Health Organization first became aware of outbreaks of the disease from reports in the London *Times* in July 1968.[15] During July and August there were scattered reports of influenza in Southeast Asia.[16] Again, initial limited establishment of the strain did not always lead to immediate explosions of influenza. The new strain reached Japan as early as July, but, interestingly, two different types of influenza virus were identified.[17] Still, the disease did not reach epidemic proportions in Japan until October. From all indications, Tokyo seems to have functioned as a slowly "smoldering" reservoir for eventual diffusion to other parts of the country.

The experience in the United States was different from some earlier episodes because of the way the disease was spreading. During the 1957 pandemic, many parts of Asia, Africa, and Europe felt the impact of influenza before the United States. Perhaps as a result of the movements of U.S. troops between Southeast Asia and America, H3N2 reached the United States before many other parts of the world. While the disease was probably already present during the summer of 1968 in the United States, the first isolated case of Hong Kong influenza virus was a Marine Corps major who had returned from Vietnam during the first week of September.[18] According to Robert Sharrar, then-chief of the Epidemic Intelligence Service of CDC, isolated cases among the civilian population appeared in widespread locations during September and early October. Those locations identified by Sharrar are shown in Figures 6.2 and 6.3. California seems to have been the first state with more widespread outbreaks, and the disease seems to have spread slowly eastward by early November 1968. The H3N2 strain seemed to have spread gradually eastward by late November to peak nationally during December. While Sharrar's reconstruction is one of the few detailed accounts during that period, it suffers from some lack of detail because of the general use of statewide data. However, the patterns of diffusion identified were based on multiple data sources for morbidity, including school and industrial absenteeism, hospital reports, and surveys of state health departments. (An alternative interpretation of the diffusion of H3N2 through the United States based on mortality data is offered later in this chapter.)

The weight of evidence seems to indicate that H3N2 spread to Britain after its arrival in the United States. The strain could have spread there from the United States, Europe, or some other part of the world. In a preliminary analysis of the pandemic, Roden demonstrated how the disease was much less severe in the United Kingdom during the winter of 1968–69 than it was in the United States.[19] In addition, influenza was a much more severe problem in the U.K. during the winter of 1967–68 than the next winter. However, events seemed to catch up with the British population, for the winter of 1969–70 was characterized by substantially more influenza mortality from H3N2.[20] This pattern was just the opposite of what happened during the 1957 pandemic.

Diffusion patterns in Eastern Europe were also different from immediately preceding pandemics. In the Soviet Union, H3N2 seems to have appeared first in December 1968 in Moscow. By January 1969, several other cities—Leningrad, Irkutsk, Dyushambe, and Tbilisi—had also emerged as diffusion epicenters.[21] By February most cities of the Soviet Union were reporting epidemics. Also, the Soviet Union had experienced a major flare-up of a variant of H2N2 during the winter of 1967–68.[22] Meanwhile, as a probable reflection of political and economic ties at that time, H3N2 seems to have spread from the Soviet Union to Czechoslovakia by January 1969.[23] As with many of the countries already mentioned, Czechoslovakia had also reported substantial influenza deaths during the winter of 1967–68.

The major impact of the arrival of H3N2 in the Southern Hemisphere was not felt until the following winter, mid-1969.[24] The disease seems to have reached South Africa by April, and outbreaks were reported in May in such widespread countries as Australia and Argentina. In almost every instance, the epidemics in the Southern Hemisphere were less severe than the epidemic initially experienced in the United States.

An Alternative Interpretation

Earliest reports may have been premature in indicating that the H3N2 pandemic was more severe in the United States than elsewhere, but many questions about what really happened in the late 1960s still remain unanswered. Over and over again, the pattern that developed within most industrialized northern-latitude countries consisted of a major epidemic of what almost certainly seems to have been H2N2 during the winter of 1967–68, followed by a less severe epidemic of H3N2 the following season. The United States also experienced a severe epidemic during the winter of 1967–68, but its seriousness was substantially overshadowed by the sheer numerical magnitude of mortality reported during the epidemic of H3N2 the following winter. The intensity of both epidemics is shown in Figure 6.4. The smooth curves represent expected and upper-threshold limits of influenza mortality as calculated by the Serfling method. The excess deaths, indicated by the sharply peaking line during the winter of 1967–68, should have served as a warning of a pending epidemic, but laboratory evidence did not agree with the statistics. Furthermore, the same thing had happened in 1956.

Influenza-mortality reporting from more than 100 of the CDC surveillance cities was examined for the period extending from midsummer to late autumn 1967 in an attempt to identify systematic geographical regularities in diffusion patterns. The major reason for such an examination was to determine if any patterns uncovered seemed to be more epidemic than endemic. Regularities could not be identified either on an urban, hierarchical basis or with regard to distance from places of origin. Actually, more than a dozen epicenters seem to have formed during that time. The patterns determined from the CDC data are also supported by influenza-mortality data derived from the then newly developed National Center for Health Statistics county computer tapes. The map in Figure 6.5 shows more than a dozen epicenters that had formed during the period. Such a pattern is indicative of both the diffusion of an established, or endemic, virus, as well as some of the spread patterns resulting from the infection of populations by H3N2.

H3N2 Influenza Reporting During September and Early October, 1968

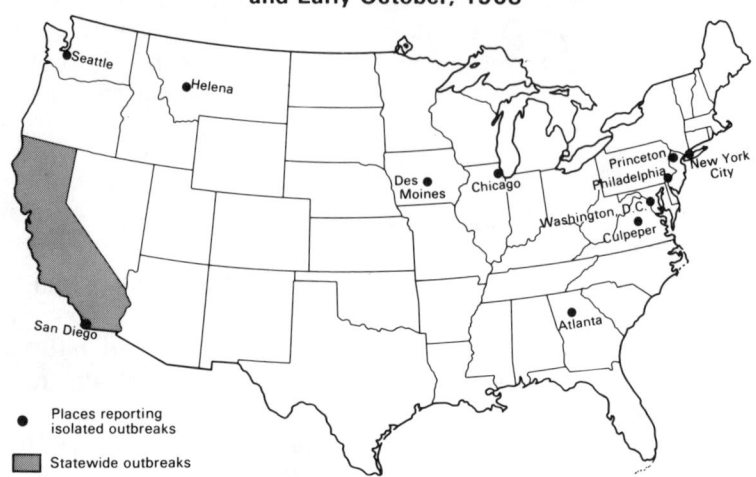

Cumulative H3N2 Outbreaks: September 28–November 9, 1968

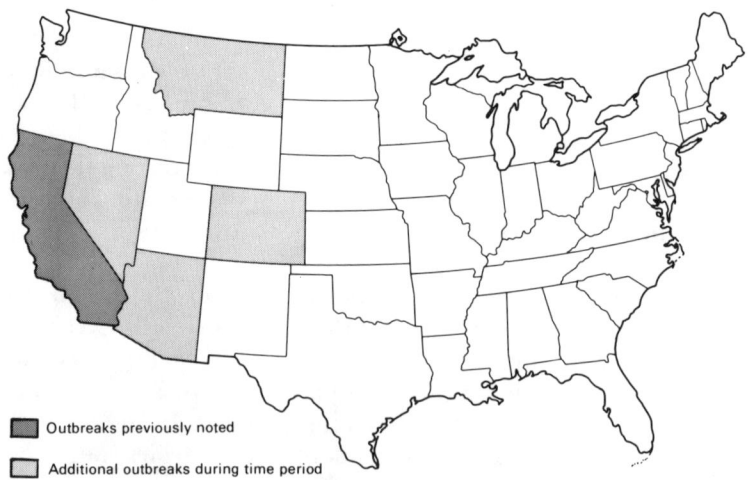

Figure 6.2. Early reports of H3N2 morbidity in the United States during the autumn of 1968.

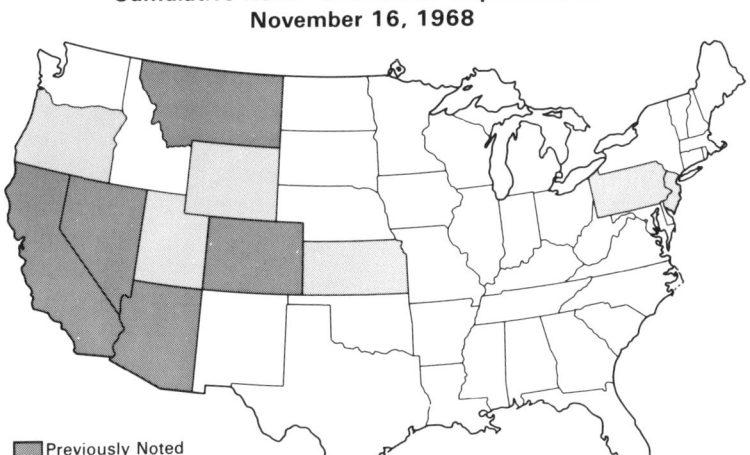

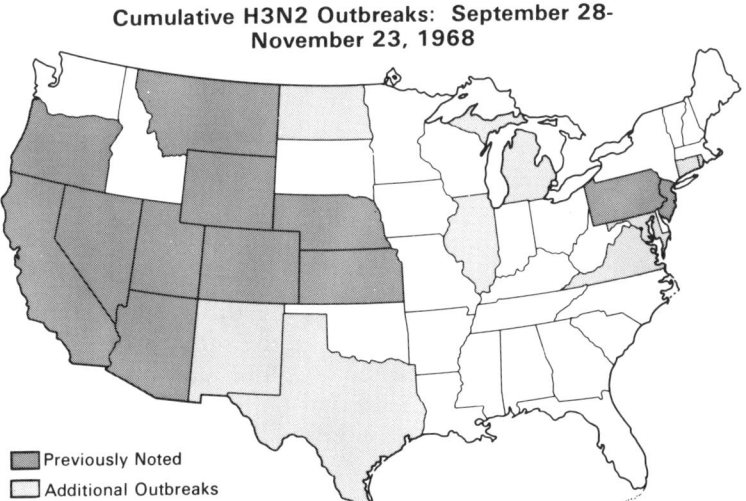

Figure 6.3. Additional autumn 1968 reports of an influenza epidemic.

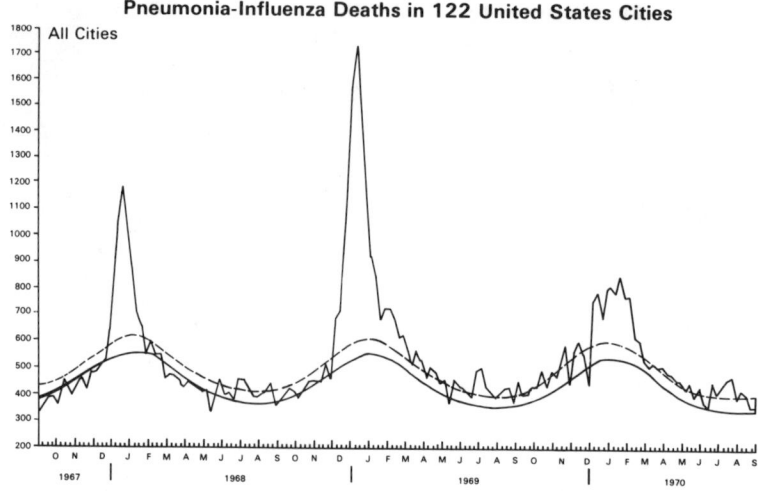

Figure 6.4. A comparison of influenza mortality in surveillance cities during winters of the late 1960s.

The next logical question to be asked is whether the diffusion patterns that resulted after the introduction of H3N2 into the U.S. population were substantially different from the early spread of the previous season. A reexamination of Figures 6.2 and 6.3 would immediately suggest that indeed a different diffusion pattern characterized the introduction of H3N2. However, when the NCHS mortality tapes are mapped in a temporal sequence, the resultant diffusion patterns continue to take the form of movement outward from multiple epicenters. Figure 6.6 shows the diffusion pathways for outbreaks that seem to have begun late in the summer of 1968. Since it is not possible to determine when and how long it took H3N2 to replace H2N2, it must be assumed that both viruses were probably contributing to the patterns in Figure 6.6. As indicated by Dowdle, the transition was gradual because of the common elements of both strains.[25] In addition, a close comparison of Figures 6.5 and 6.6 suggests that many places that formed epicenters in 1968 were not points of origin for diffusion the previous season. This association is characteristic of some of the rhythmic pulsations that take place when similar strains move within and among regions from one season to the next.[26]

There is, of course, also the remote possibility that the initial transformations of virus types actually began first within interior portions of the North American continent. Following such logic, the changing strains were further carried to Southeast Asia and then Hong Kong, whereupon the new strain subsequently diffused to the

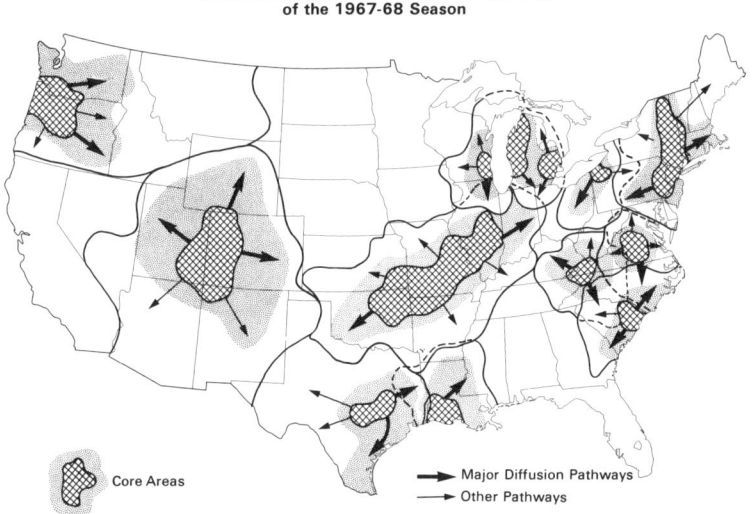

Core Areas and Diffusion Pathways for Primary
Outbreaks of Influenza During the Beginning
of the 1967-68 Season

Core Areas

→ Major Diffusion Pathways
→ Other Pathways

Figure 6.5. Widespread epicenters of the 1967–68 epidemic of the prevailing strain a year or so before the introduction of a new strain. As with past similar circumstances, no new form of influenza had yet been recognized.

United States and other countries. Such a possibility is probably not realistic, but we are still no more sure of the origins of the 1968 pandemic than those of 1918.

Assuming the conventional wisdom that H3N2 did spread from the Orient, it is possible to suggest patterns of diffusion from the CDC surveillance-cities mortality data. Keeping in mind the accelerated mortality rates during the 1967–68 season, it seems that influenza waned during April 1968. Expected rates as determined by Serfling's model were attained during the summer of 1968, but there were several flare-ups of note (see Fig. 6.4). Indications are that while influenza deaths continued to wane during May, as shown in Figure 6.7, minor outbreaks of influenza occurred in Chicago, New York, and many other major cities during June. Reporting declined again during July (Fig. 6.8), only to increase in a major fashion in August. The pattern of reporting in Figure 6.8 strongly suggests that by then H3N2 was well seeded. As indicated by influenza workers during the late 1960s, the disease then seems truly to have "smoldered." The patterns shown in Figures 6.9, 6.10, and 6.11 help explain this phenomenon. In September 1968 influenza reporting was substantially less than during August. Cities that registered increases in mortality were in fact widely scattered. As the epidemic began to strengthen during October and November, epidemic thresholds were

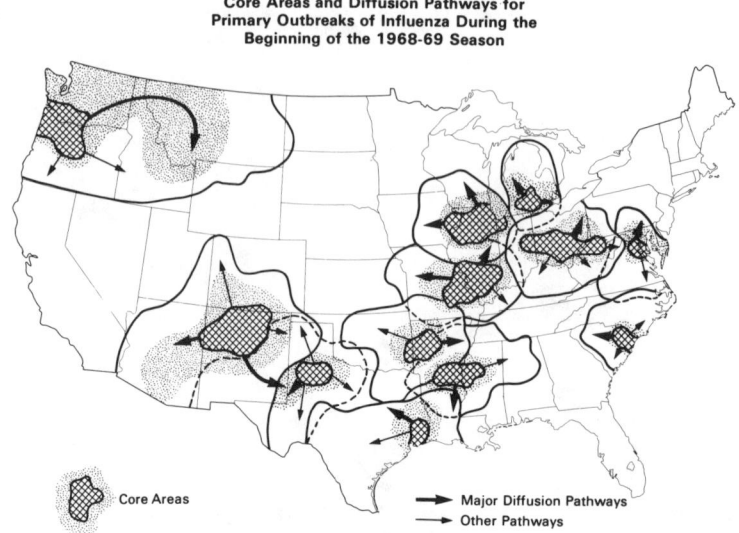

**Core Areas and Diffusion Pathways for
Primary Outbreaks of Influenza During the
Beginning of the 1968-69 Season**

Core Areas   ➡ Major Diffusion Pathways
                  → Other Pathways

Figure 6.6. Possible outbreak epicenters of H3N2 during autumn 1968.

exceeded. Sharrar's earlier suggestions of the gradual spread of influenza from west to east cannot be substantiated by the CDC city mortality reporting patterns. Instead, the disease seems to have spread outward from several urban centers simultaneously, as indicated by the NCHS data. The strongest indications of this kind of diffusion show up in the December 1968 mapping. Those cities where influenza mortality had already peaked for the season are indicated by solid circles. Then, in January 1969, influenza mortality peaked in most surveillance cities, and by February the disease had begun to wane.

A Sampling of Locations

Temporal reporting of epidemic-level increases and maximum impact of the disease seem to agree with the preceding mapping of P&I deaths in urban areas in the United States. Such indications are included in studies of the epidemic developed for a variety of reasons and using different kinds of test populations. For example, in one of the most interesting analyses of the appearance of H3N2 in Hong Kong, researchers from America, Britain, and China combined efforts and concluded that the new strain first appeared in Hong Kong in July 1968.[27] The disease spread rapidly to all age groups. Continuous laboratory testing upheld the notion that the new strain had some

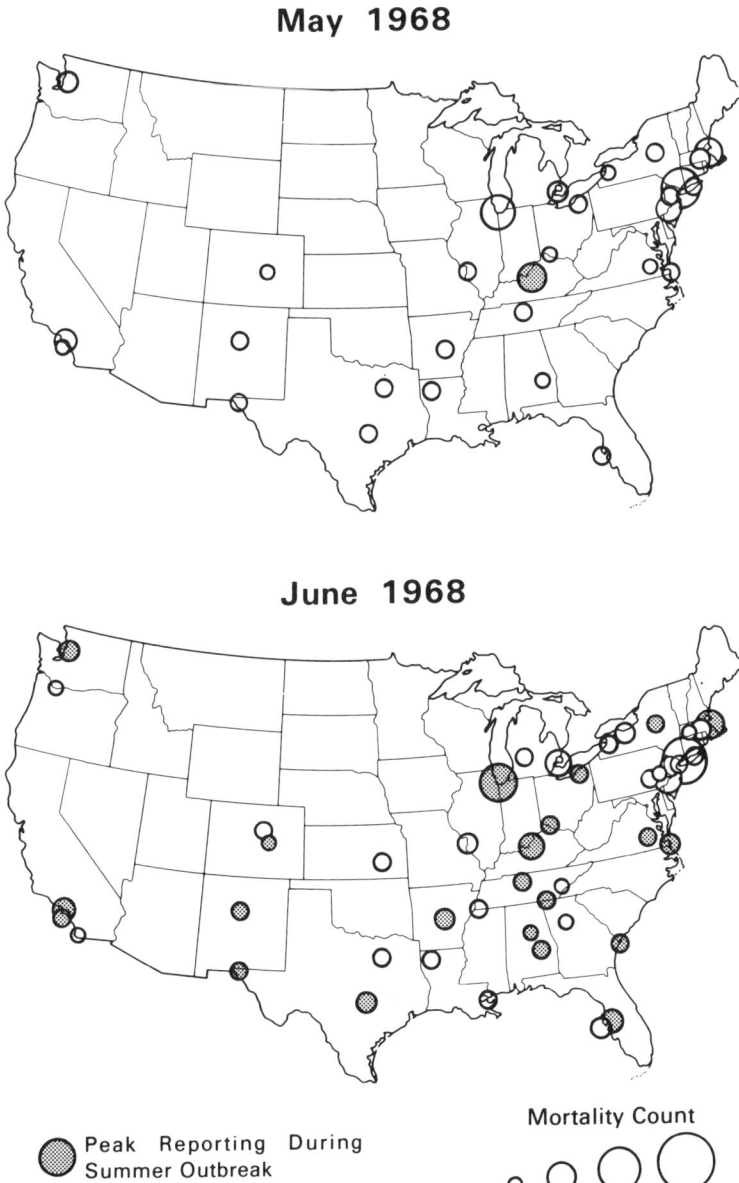

Figure 6.7. Unusual influenza mortality reporting during the early summer of 1968.

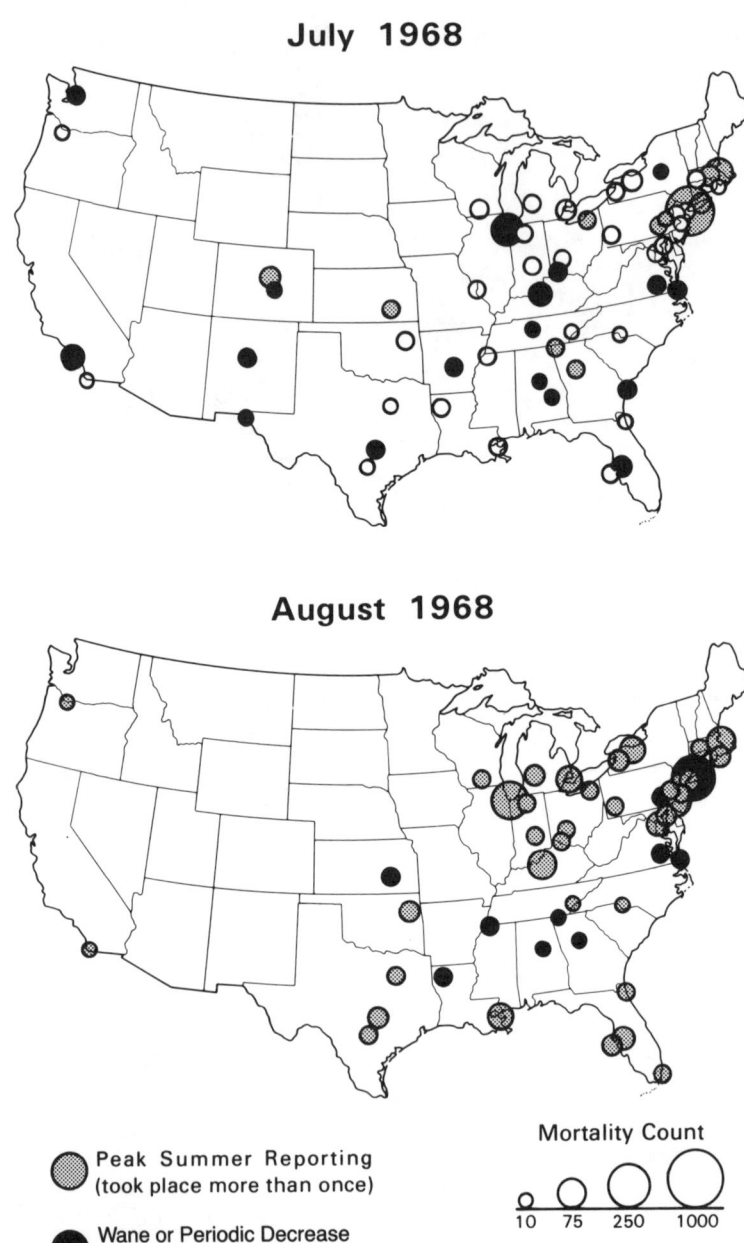

Figure 6.8. Influenza mortality during the summer of 1968 continued to be unusual, with widespread oscillations in numbers of flu-related deaths.

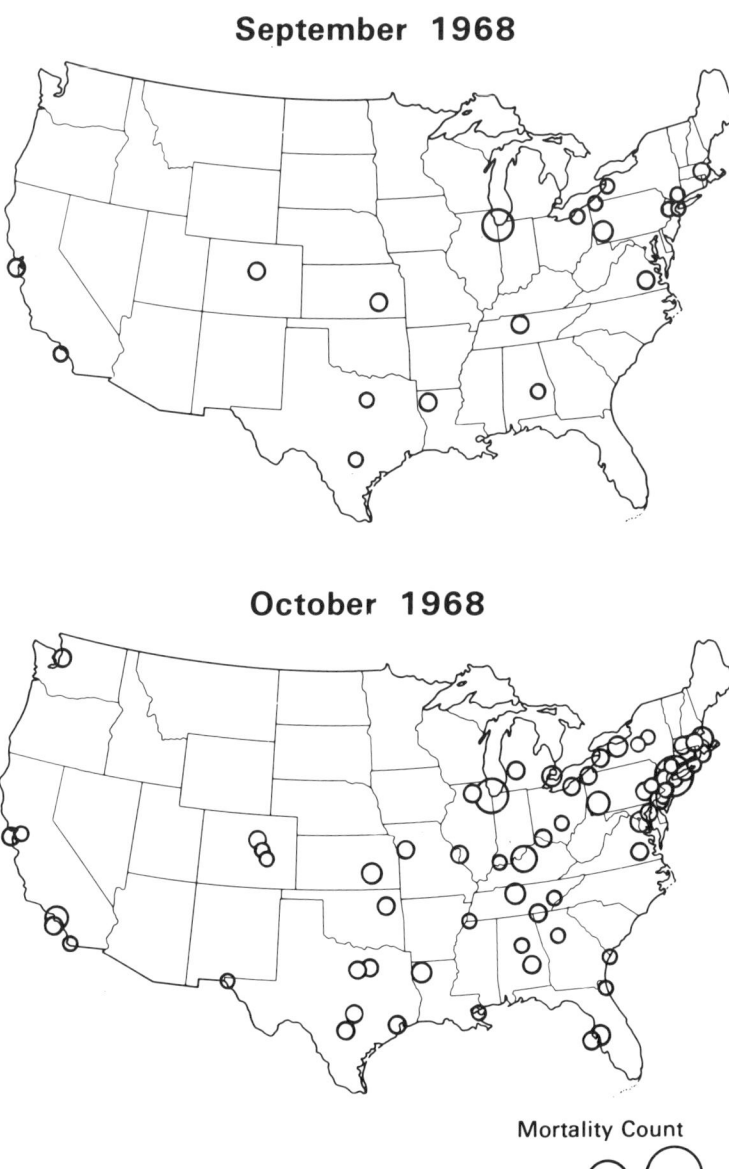

Figure 6.9. Influenza mortality had waned by September 1968, and the "smoldering" period seemed to be over. As H2N2, or Hong Kong influenza, emerged as the prevailing strain, multiple epicenters had formed.

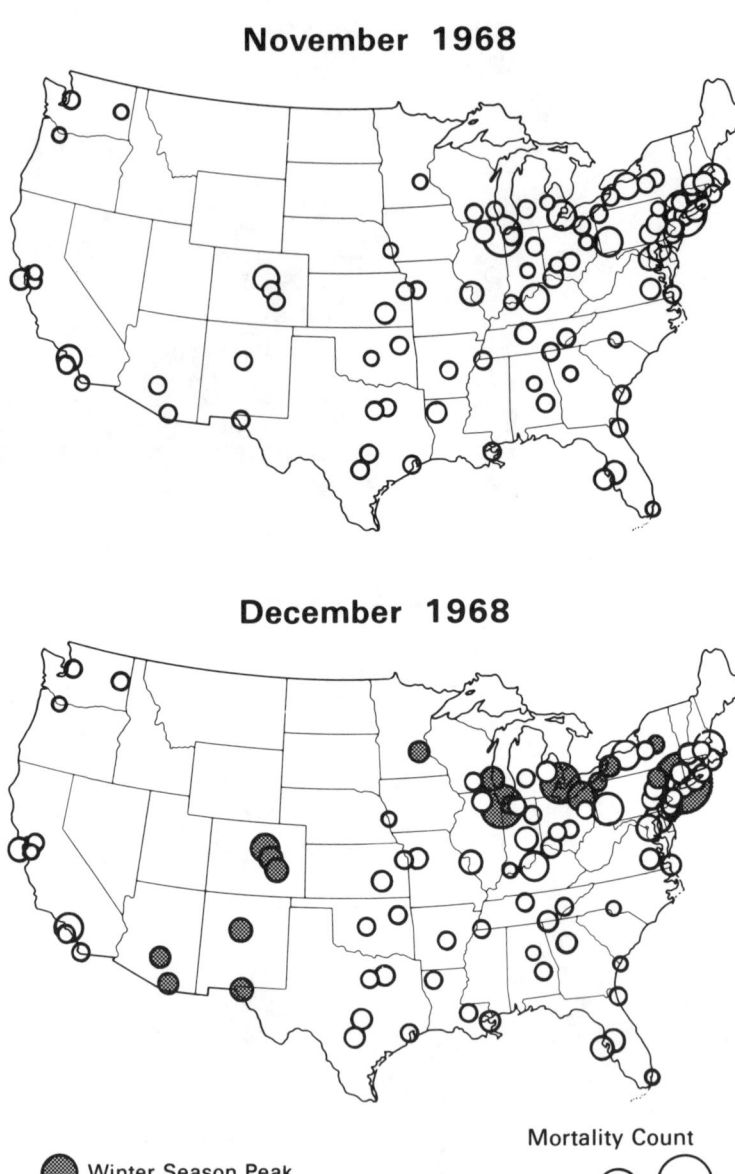

Figure 6.10. Mortality reporting during late 1968.

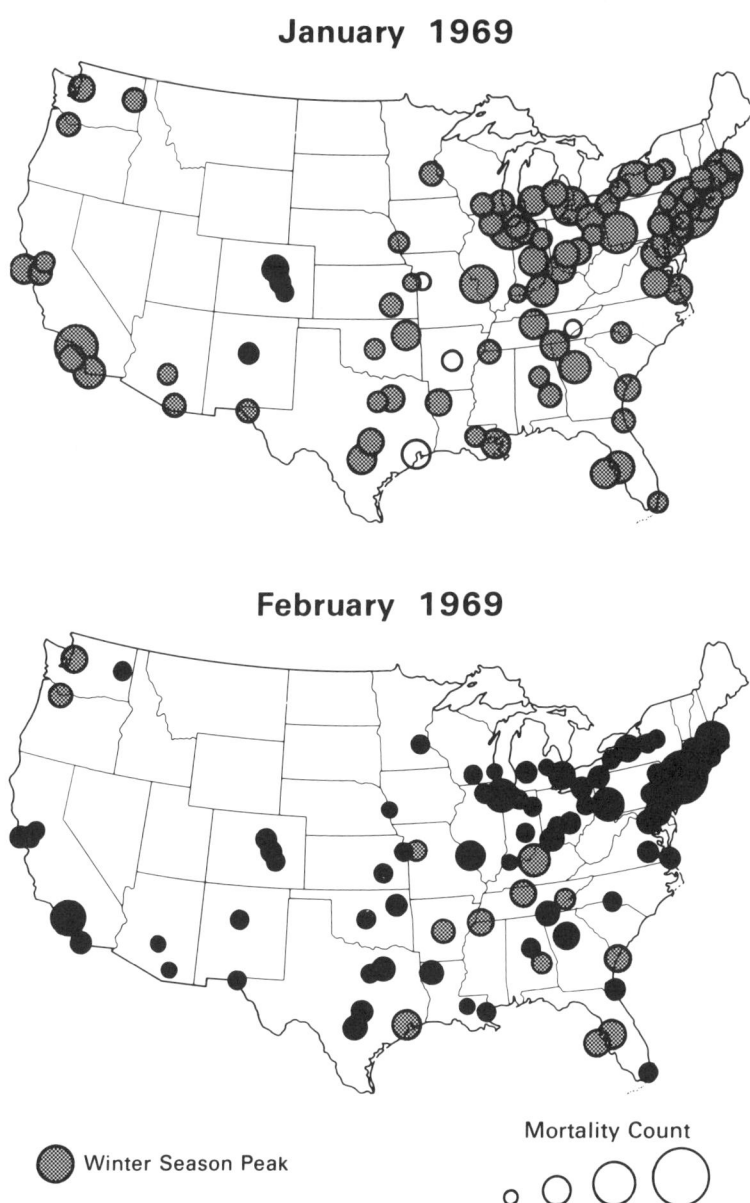

Figure 6.11. By January and February of 1969, H3N2 had peaked and waned within most CDC surveillance cities.

genetic similarities to the previous strain, but there were sufficient differences that immunity to H2N2 did not guarantee immunity to H3N2.[28]

There is less agreement, primarily because of the nature of H3N2 seeding, on just when the new strain first appeared in the United States than there is about when temporal peaking actually occurred. The transfer of the well-known influenza Virus Watch from New York to Seattle during the mid-1960s offered an excellent opportunity to observe important temporal aspects of several different influenza variants that spread through the population in the late 1960s.[29] Primarily concerned with the influenza threat to children, researchers from the Seattle Virus Watch also were able to depict temporal trends. According to Hall, Cooney, and Fox, H3N2 was introduced to Seattle's population in September 1968, but it did not spread until November—again, the smoldering effect. As with most parts of the country, the introductory H3N2 epidemic peaked during January 1969 (see Fig. 6.13). Since the Seattle Virus Watch was also concerned with the prevalence of influenza B within the youthful population, it is important to note that the documentation of the epidemic of 1967–68 (H2N2) showed little evidence of Influenza B; but there was an epidemic of B within the youthful population at the same time that H3N2 was affecting most age groups.

Related studies in other cities offer strong support for the temporal relationships depicted in Figures 6.9, 6.10, and 6.11. A study by the Milwaukee Health Department indicates that while influenza did not officially peak nationally until mid-January 1969, the epidemic had reached some of its highest proportions by mid-December 1968.[30] In addition to reported excess P&I mortality, the Milwaukee study used three new measures: (1) laboratory-confirmed cases; (2) work absenteeism; and (3) hospital admissions. Such careful studies offer strong support for the use of multiple measures of temporal aspects of influenza during an epidemic in selected locations. Conversely, general temporal aspects of the disease under epidemic conditions can be identified by carefully scrutinizing hospital admissions for respiratory ailments. A study of Memphis hospitals during the 1968–69 pandemic also confirms the pattern of spatial diffusion shown in Figures 6.9 to 6.11.[31]

Speculations on Equine Influenza and Other Connections

The H3N2 pandemic resulted in a flurry of research in influenza epidemiology. Although new hypotheses about different strains of influenza emerged, most research continued along the lines that had been established prior to 1968. Also, most conventional twentieth-century approaches to influenza research that had developed prior to the H3N2 pandemic, including viral replacement, classification of viruses, animal influenza, vaccine efficacy, and pathogenesis, continued into the 1970s, even though Hoyle's extensive explanation of these trends, along with an even more extensive bibliography, was published in 1968, *before* the H3N2 pandemic. Those accounts nonetheless shed considerable light on the problem of viral replacement,[32] and the H3N2 pandemic did not lead to any changes in such thinking. One of the most intriguing lines of research (and speculation to some extent) that surfaced after the H3N2 pandemic followed the logic that the 1968 pandemic of human influenza was caused by a virus related to the agent causing influenza in horses, and there was also a possible connection between equine influenza and flu in humans in the 1870s.

The equine, or "horse flu," association was in effect more than simple speculation, and it influenced the efforts of a number of influenza researchers in the late 1960s. Probably the first indication of a virological connection was that noted in an article in *Lancet* on influenza in Hong Kong during July 1968.[33] While it had long been suggested, following the logic of Shope and others, that some animals can serve as repositories for different strains of influenza, research during the 1960s could now suggest several minor antigenic similarities. In fact, human volunteers had been successfully infected with equine influenza several years before the H3N2 pandemic. One of the most noteworthy studies was accomplished using prison inmates.[34] The rationale for these studies was that the equine influenza agent, first identified in 1956 in Europe and in 1963 in America, had caused some historical epizootics prior to human influenza epidemics. Some researchers therefore thought that epizootics of "horse flu" might lead in subsequent seasons to human influenza pandemics caused by newly emergent or recycled strains. In fact, equine influenza seems to have circulated both before and after the more recent human H3N2 and H2N2 pandemics, as well as before and after some late nineteenth-century epidemics.[35] A 1969 study released by the World Health Organization concluded that there may have been an outbreak of H3N2 in the late nineteenth century, but that equine influenzalike viruses may have prevailed in man before the pandemic of 1889–90.[36] Subsequent recombination in some form could have led to an outbreak of human influenza in 1900, and if that is the case, it could have recurred in 1968. Such studies eventually led to a clarification in procedures used with systems of influenza virus nomenclature and the relationship between genetic recombinations and influenza vaccines.[37]

Comparisons with the Conventional Wisdom

Several aspects of the appearance of influenza strains other than the prevailing types seem to have been reinforced by the pandemic of 1968. Vaccines continuously under improvement during the 1960s[38] had little initial effect against the disease until a vaccine was developed against H3N2.[39] One strain (H2N2) was indeed replaced by another, and the emergent strain may have circulated within the human population before. The new strain seems to have originated in China. There was also a partial association with an animal form of influenza.

Aspects of the geography of influenza in the late 1960s, however, hardly correspond to many of the gross generalizations found in the literature about the spread of the disease. For example, such observations as "In 1968, the disease once again swept the country from west to east" are unfounded. On the other hand, explanations tied to seeding and subsequent eruption from multiple epicenters can be supported. One important and possibly unique aspect of the H3N2 pandemic is the extensive activity of a probably drifting variant of H2N2 internationally during the winter of 1967–68. In addition, that phenomenon may have had a dampening effect on influenza the next

**Regions with Highest Reporting During Epidemics:
1967-68 (H2N2) and 1968-69 (H3N2)**

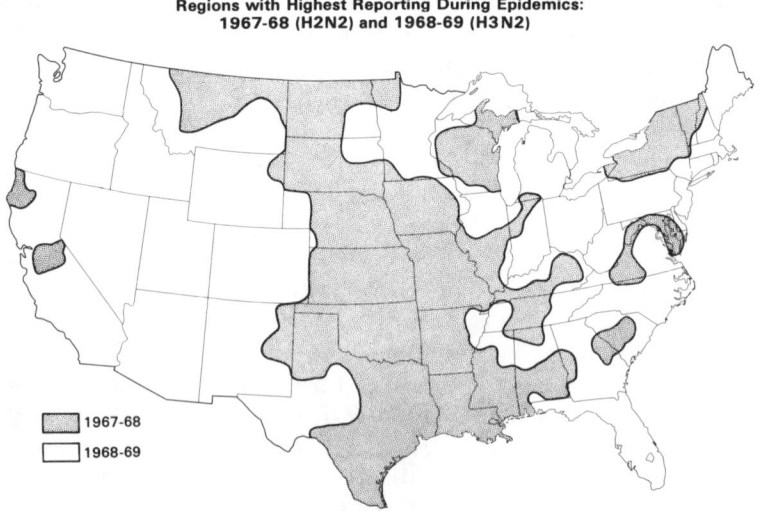

1967-68
1968-69

Figure 6.12. This map helps to clear up some of the confusion about influenza strains during the late 1960s because it shows how there were actually more deaths due to a prevailing strain in central parts of the country during the winter before the introduction of a new virus. Since there was so much "smoldering" during the summer of 1968, one can't help but wonder if "Hong Kong" influenza didn't originate in Nebraska, Kansas, or Missouri.

winter.[40] Also, for some still-unknown reason, the pandemic of H3N2 struck the United States with more impact initially than in some other parts of the world. But even so, not all parts of the United States reported more influenza during the winter of 1968–69 than during the previous season. The map in Figure 6.12, based on NCHS data tapes, reveals that county health departments in many parts of the country, especially in interior areas, actually reported increased influenza mortality during the winter before the H3N2 pandemic.[41] All indications are that most of these deaths were somehow associated with H2N2, since the new strain had not yet surfaced in China.

In keeping with what was "expected," there were at least two waves of the H3N2 pandemic (see Fig. 6.13). Influenza mortality waned substantially, as indicated by both CDC and NCHS reports during the early 1970s, but minor outbreaks occurred during the winters of 1971–72 and 1972–73. By the mid-1970s, influenza seemed again to increase gradually, but no new strain was either identified or expected. Then, not to the surprise of those who had long held the notion that influenza viruses can be transmitted from humans to animals and back again in varied forms, the inevitable seems to have happened. The danger, however, was not an equine influenza that is somehow related to H3N2. The disease threat that suddenly appeared in early 1976 was *swine* influenza, the agent that may have caused the 1918–19 pandemic. The time had finally come for a

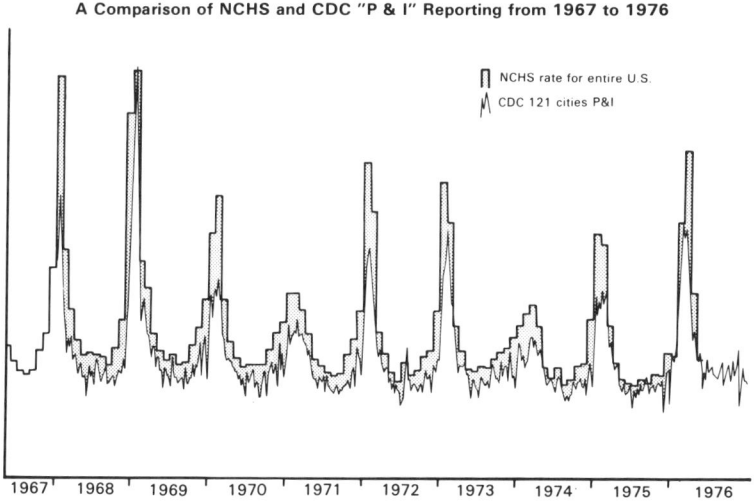

A Comparison of NCHS and CDC "P & I" Reporting from 1967 to 1976

∏ NCHS rate for entire U.S.

∧ CDC 121 cities P&I

1967 1968 1969 1970 1971 1972 1973 1974 1975 1976

Figure 6.13. This comparison of influenza deaths as reported by two different federal agencies suggests that the disease could have been a much more serious public health threat than initially thought during the winter of 1967–68.

nationally coordinated effort to prevent, or at least diminish, the impact of future epidemics.

Notes

1. C. H. Andrewes, "Observations on Hong Kong/A2 Influenza Origins," *Proceedings, Royal Society of Medicine* 64 (1968).
2. Robert E. Serfling, I. Sherman, and W. J. Housworth, "Excess Pneumonia-Influenza Mortality by Age and Sex in Three Major A2 Epidemics, United States, 1957–58, 1960 and 1963," *American Journal of Epidemiology* 86, (1967), pp. 433–41.
3. Robert E. Serfling, "Methods of Current Statistical Analysis of Excess Pneumonia-Influenza Deaths," *Public Health Reports* 78 (1963), pp. 494–506.
4. Ibid., p. 500.
5. Theodore C. Eikhoff and Roslyn Q. Robinson, "Influenza Surveillance, United States, 1960," *Public Health Reports* 76 (1961), pp. 1099–1106.
6. Yates Trotter, Jr., Frederick Dunn, Robert H. Drachman, Donald A. Henderson, Mario Pizzi, and Alexander Langmuir, "Asian Influenza in the United States, 1957–1958," *American Journal of Hygiene* 70 (1959), pp. 34–50.
7. Jere Housworth and Alexander Langmuir, "Excess Mortality from Epidemic Influenza, 1957–1966," *American Journal of Epidemiology* 100 (1974), pp. 40–48.
8. Theodore Eikhoff, Ida L. Sherman, and Robert E. Serfling, "Observations on Excess Mortality Associated with Epidemic Influenza," *Journal of the American Medical Association* 176 (June 3, 1961), pp. 104–10.
9. Ibid., p. 109.
10. Alexander D. Langmuir and Jere Housworth, "A Critical Evaluation of Influenza Surveillance," *Bulletin, World Health Organization* 41 (1969), pp. 393–98.
11. Edwin D. Kilbourne, "Future Influenza Vaccines and the Use of Genetic Recombinants," *Bulletin, World Health Organization* 41 (1969), pp. 643–45.
    Maurice R. Hilleman, "The Roles of Early Alert and of Adjuvant in the Control of Hong Kong Influenza by Vaccines," *Bulletin, World Health Organization* 41 (1969), pp. 623–28.
12. J. C. McDonald, "Influenza in Canada," *Canadian Medical Association Journal* 97 (1967), pp. 522–27.
13. Hedio Fukumi, "The Meaning and Appearance of Hong Kong Influenza," *Archives of Environmental Health* 21 (1970), pp. 304–6.
14. W. Charles Cockburn, P. J. Delon, and W. Ferreira, "Origin and Progress of the 1968–69 Hong Kong Influenza Epidemic," *Bulletin, World Health Organization* 41 (1969), pp. 345–48.
15. Ibid., p. 345.
16. Marion T. Coleman, Walter R. Dowdle, Helio G. Pereira, Geoffrey C. Schild, and W. K. Chang, "The Hong Kong/68 Influenza A2 Variant," *Lancet* 1 (1968), pp. 1384–86.
17. Hideo Fukumi, "Summary Report on Hong Kong Influenza in Japan," *Bulletin, World Health Organization* 41 (1969), pp. 353–59.
18. Robert G. Sharrar, "National Influenza Experience in the USA," *Bulletin, World Health Organization* 41 (1969), pp. 361–66.
19. A. T. Roden, "National Experience with Hong Kong Influenza in the United Kingdom, 1968–69," *Bulletin, World Health Organization* 41 (1969), pp. 375–80.
20. Rosemary E. Clifford, J. W. G. Smith, Hilary Tillett, and Patricia J. Wherry, "Excess Mortality Associated with Influenza in England and Wales," *International Journal of Epidemiology* 6 (1977), pp. 115–28.
21. L. Ja. Zakstelskaja, N. A. Evstigneeva, V. A. Isachenko, S. Ph. Shenderovitch, and V. A. Efimova, "Influenza in the USSR: New Antigenic Variation A2/Hong Kong/1/68 and Its Possible Precursors," *American Journal of Epidemiology* 90 (1969), pp. 400–405.

22. V. M. Zdanov and I. V. Antonova, "The Hong Kong Virus Epidemic in the USSR," *Bulletin, World Health Organization* 41 (1969), pp. 381–86.
23. D. Fedova, M. Drasnar, P. Strnad, J. Vobecky, J. Jelinek, E. Svandova, M. Sampalik, and L. Syrucek, "Hong Kong Influenza in Czechoslovakia, 1969," *Bulletin, World Health Organization* 41 (1969), pp. 367–73.
24. E. L. Buescher, T. J. Smith, and I. H. Zachary. "Experience with Hong Kong Influenza in Tropical Areas," *Bulletin, World Health Organization* 41 (1969), pp. 387–91.
25. Walter R. Dowdle, "Influenza: Epidemic Patterns and Antigenic Variation," in Philip Selby, ed., *Influenza: Virus, Vaccines and Strategy* (London and New York: Academic Press. 1976), pp. 17–21.
26. Alexander Langmuir, Donald A. Henderson, and Robert E. Serfling, "The Epidemiological Basis for the Control of Influenza," *American Journal of Public Health* 54 (1964), pp. 563–71.
27. Coleman et al., "The Hong Kong/68 Influenza A2 Variant."
28. W. K. Chang, "National Influenza Experience in Hong Kong, 1968," *Bulletin, World Health Organization* 41 (1969), pp. 349–51.
29. Carrie E. Hall, Marion K. Cooney, and John P. Fox, "The Seattle Virus Watch," *American Journal of Epidemiology* 98 (1973), pp. 365–80.
30. Frank F. Piraino, Edwin M. Brown, and Edward R. Krumbiegel, "Outbreak of Hong Kong Influenza in Milwaukee, Winter of 1968–69," *Public Health Reports* 85 (1970), pp. 140–50.
31. Alan L. Bisno, John P. Griffin, Kenneth A. Van Epps, Harvey B. Neill, and Michael W. Rytel, "Pneumonia and Hong Kong Influenza: A Prospective Study of the 1968–1969 Epidemic," *American Journal of the Medical Sciences* 261 (1971), pp. 251–63.
32. L. Hoyle, *The Influenza Viruses* (New York: Springer-Verlag, 1968).
33. Coleman et al., "The Hong Kong/68 Influenza A2 Variant."
34. Julius A. Kasel, Robert H. Alford, and Vernon Knight, "Experimental Infection of Human Volunteers with Equine Influenza Virus," *Nature* 206 (1965), pp. 41–43.
35. F. M. Davenport, E. Minuse, A. V. Hennessy, and T. Francis, Jr., "Interpretations of Influenza Antibody Patterns of Man," *Bulletin, World Health Organization* 41 (1969), pp. 453–60.
36. Robert H. Alford, Julius A. Kasel, James R. Lehrich, and Vernon Knight, "Human Responses to Experimental Infection with Influenza A/Equi 2 Virus," *American Journal of Epidemiology* 86 (1967), pp. 185–92.
37. Bela Tumova and Bernard C. Easterday, "Relationships of Envelope Antigens of Animal Influenza Viruses to Human A2 Influenza Strains Isolated in the Years 1957–68," *Bulletin, World Health Organization* 41 (1969), pp. 429–35.
38. William H. Stuart, Bruce Dull, Ladine H. Newton, James L. McQueen, and Eugene R. Schiff, "Evaluation of Monovalent Influenza Vaccine in a Retirement Community During the Epidemic of 1965–1966," *Journal of the American Medical Association* 209 (July 14, 1969), pp. 232–38.
39. William M. Marine and Wilton Workman, "Hong Kong Influenza Immunologic Recapitulation," *American Journal of Epidemiology* 90 (1969), pp. 406–15.
40. Dowdle, "Influenza: Epidemic Patterns and Antigen Variations."
41. These observations are based on extensive processing of data tapes from the National Center for Health Statistics.

7

Reflections on the "Swine Flu" Scare of 1976

By the late 1970s we had entered an exciting scientific era because of the remarkable innovations in microcomputational technology. Many of these new technologies led to tremendous strides in methods of accumulating medical information, and this accumulation ultimately led to improved disease control and prevention strategies. It therefore seemed disappointingly paradoxical that presumably newer forms of infectious diseases continued to lead to unprecedented public health hazards. Herpes appeared to be rampant, and the high death rate of those suffering from acquired immune deficiency syndrome (AIDS) presented an awesome specter that was a direct challenge to the improved disease-treatment efforts. Other examples of the unexplained outbreak of lethal infectious diseases included the Legionnaire's Disease episode of 1976 and the sudden appearance of "swine flu" at Fort Dix, New Jersey, earlier the same year.

The story of the swine-influenza outbreak and the subsequent public reaction in the United States, while dramatic because it represented a major change in the prevailing conservative public health policies, initially seemed to be as perplexing as the sudden proliferation of infectious diseases. Many public health and medical researchers believed that the type of swine influenza that was recovered from human victims during the January 1976 outbreak at Fort Dix was closely related to the agent that caused more than 500,000 deaths in the United States during the 1918–19 pandemic. In response to this emergency, a nationwide inoculation program was instituted. Opposition to the program surfaced immediately, however, and congressional support gradually diminished during the first six months of 1976. The sudden outbreak of a respiratory disease at an American Legion convention in Philadelphia in July 1976—it was six months before a bacterial agent was isolated—resulted in another phase of public alarm.[1] Proponents of the influenza inoculation program now

This chapter was adapted from Gerald F. Pyle, "Spatial Perspectives on Influenza Acceptance and Policy," *Economic Geography* 60 (1984), pp. 273–93.

had the necessary support, and distribution of vaccines to the public officially began in October 1976.

This chapter has two major purposes: (1) to analyze spatial aspects of influenza diffusion before and after the national inoculation program in an attempt to develop an understanding of its geographical impact; and (2) to compare spatial similarities and differences in the actual acceptance of the vaccines so that such information might be used in support of any future related programs. Prior to this analysis, only state-level inoculation data have been used for comparative purposes.[2] The chapter will also examine the relationship between city size and inoculation acceptance patterns in order to test conventional views about diffusion. Both anticipated and unexpected influenza patterns prior to the inoculation program that began in October 1976 will be examined, followed by a geographical comparison of the dissemination of the vaccine over the next several months. Influenza-diffusion patterns after the inoculation program will be explained, and some general recommendations will be made with reference to the spatial aspects of related, future programs.

While the modern era in influenza research and control actually began with the discovery of the virus in 1933, it was not until antibiotics and influenza vaccines were developed that researchers posited the notion of ten-year cycles.[3] Since viruses cannot be contained by antibiotics, we began to learn more about changes in the nature of the influenza agent when the 1947 virus was introduced into the American population.[4] This strain prevailed for about a decade, but the vaccine developed from that virus was useless against the 1957 (Asian) influenza. It is also of special interest with reference to organized inoculation efforts that the 1957 strain was first detected during the spring of 1957, and since the "heavy" influenza season normally begins in the autumn with a winter peak, the necessary six-month lead time was available to develop a new vaccine. A vaccine was developed, but there was only minimal support for a public inoculation program. The official national public policy at that time was that the private sector—physicians and hospitals—could easily deal with the problem. A federal inoculation program then might have saved thousands of lives.[5] A similar set of circumstances seemed to prevail when "Hong Kong" influenza surfaced in 1968.[6] The 1957 Asian virus seemed to disappear from the population, as had the earlier 1947 virus. The death toll from the 1968 virus in the United States was lower than that of the decade before, probably because the virus that replaced the prevailing strain was characterized by a less complex genetic change and was less virulent.[7] Because of this, many health-policy makers felt no need for an inoculation program. Conversely, the ten-year periodicity of epidemic influenza cycles indeed seems to have become established.

During the early to mid-1970s, extensive research had been accomplished with influenza viruses in the United States and abroad.[8] Increased knowledge of the nature of influenza viruses and propensities toward both genetic drift and shift could be incorporated into a standardized international influenza-nomenclature system. The basis for this system as proposed by the World Health Organization consisted of the relationship between the hemagglutinin (H) and neuraminidase (N) spikes on the outer shell of the influenza virus, as well as some components within the protein core.[9] Thus, the 1947 virus is now called H1N1, that which surfaced in 1957 is H2N2 (a double genetic shift), and the 1968 virus has become known as H3N2. Initially within this revised nomenclature system, most viruses identified prior to 1947 were labeled H0N1, the exception being the Hsw1N1 virus (swine flu) that *may have* caused the 1918–20 pandemic. Later, after the inoculation program of 1976, the Center for Disease Control in Atlanta proposed that the H0N1, H1N1, and Hsw1N1 strains were sufficiently related biologically to be considered of the same general viral strain. That change in nomenclature shed some light on attempts to explain the influenza outbreaks in the United States in the late 1970s.

The Fort Dix Paradox and Related Events

Given this backlog of information, it was not surprising that a new strain of influenza was expected by the late 1970s. According to Kilbourne, the ten-year viral-replacement cycle is based on the relationship between immune and susceptible populations.[10] As immunity to a strain of influenza virus increases over time within a population and resistance builds up, new strains emerge and new epidemics or pandemics result. Then immunity levels build up again before the sequence is repeated. Many health professionals thought that this sequence was repeating itself during the early part of 1976 with the outbreak of swine flu at Fort Dix, New Jersey. In mid-January 1976, a large number of cases of respiratory disease were reported at Fort Meade, Maryland, and at Fort Dix.[11] Throat cultures from Fort Dix were identified as the prevailing H3N2 virus or an unknown virus. In mid-February the Center for Disease Control confirmed that the unknown virus was swine influenza. An emergency meeting was held to discuss these findings and to make plans to develop a vaccine. Quantities of the Fort Dix virus were delivered to vaccine manufacturers, but for some reason they did not grow well in their labs. By late February there were reports of swine influenza in humans from Minnesota, Wisconsin, Pennsylvania, Virginia, and Mississippi, but the disease was apparently not spreading rapidly within the population. In March the CDC recommended that the Ford Administration ask Congress for $134 million for a national inoculation program. Since no attempt was made for such a program in 1957 or 1968, and given that the six-month lead time necessary to develop a vaccine was available prior to an expected high influenza death rate during the 1976–77 winter, the stage seemed to be set for an unprecedented program. Congressional hearings were held in late March to determine the feasibility of such a program.

The other perplexing circumstance that occurred during the first several months of 1976 was the exceptionally high number of deaths attributed to influenza-pneumonia. In addition, a clearly defined pattern of outward diffusion from January to March from the northeastern United States can be identified. Actually, there were no indications during the late fall and early winter of the 1976–77 season that an outbreak of influenza would become severe. However, Philadelphia's January 1976 influenza deaths were reported as double the January average for the past decade. While this was not initially the case with New York City, by February New York had also begun to report influenza deaths substantially higher than its ten-year February average. The spatial extent of the problem can be partially ascertained by examining Figures 7.1 and 7.2. These four maps show which surveillance cities reported either one and one-half or two times the ten-year-average number of cases during January, February, March, and April 1976. Influenza reporting was exceptionally high during this period, but the virus was not identified as swine influenza. Instead, the reporting has been attributed to a combination of a number of viruses related to the prevailing H3N2 strain.[12] Awareness of a possible influenza epidemic may have led to increased identifications of deaths attributed to the disease by public health workers on the lookouts for its occurrence. Regardless of the circumstances, an epidemic appears to have begun in the Philadelphia–New Jersey–Greater New York area. By February, at the same time the swine flu virus was identified by the CDC, the spring epidemic gathered momentum and spread from its megalopolis core westward toward the Mississippi River and into the Southeast. An almost classic diffusion pattern seems to have emerged.

The circles in Figures 7.1 and 7.2 depict the numerical range of cases, thus indicating the magnitude of the problem initially in the Northeast and then in other areas of the country. By March the epidemic seems to have exploded in the West. While it is conjectured here that the latter pattern is the result of hierarchical diffusion based on city size, it is also possible to obtain moderate distance-decay associations for the 51 surveillance cities east of the 100th meridian. Since rates can be a stronger indication of influenza intensity during

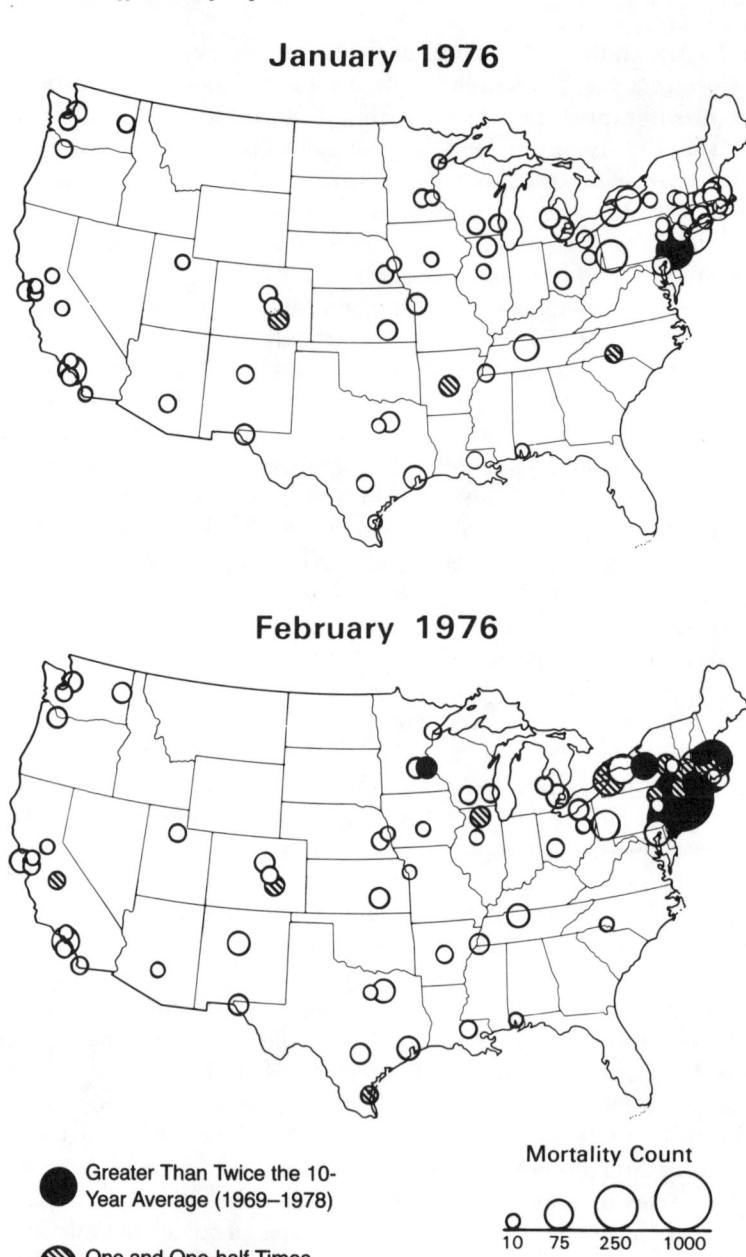

January 1976

February 1976

Greater Than Twice the 10-
Year Average (1969–1978)

One and One-half Times
the 10-Year Average
(1969–1978)

Mortality Count

10   75   250   1000

Figure 7.1. These maps show how an unexpected outbreak of a prevailing strain of influenza originated along the Eastern Seaboard during the winter before the reintroduction of H1N1.

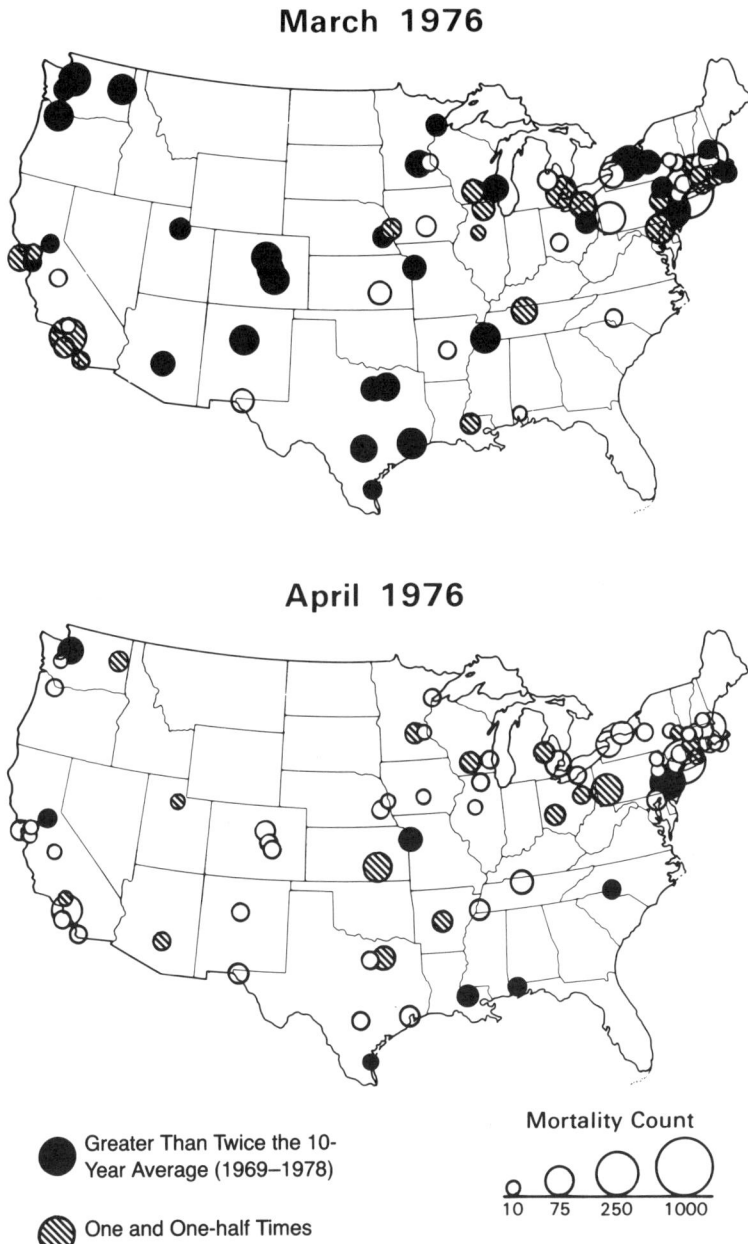

Figure 7.2. By March 1976, an epidemic of H3N2 had swept through urban areas, and by April reporting had declined.

an epidemic, they were compared in a negative exponential regression, using distance from Philadelphia (the presumed outbreak center) as the independent variable for the eastern cities. Significant pairwise correlations were derived in that manner: January, $-.385$; February, $-.589$; and March, $-.357$. Hierarchical effects can also be identified before March in the Southwest and West by comparing rates and distance during February. Three distinct clusters are shown in Figure 7.3. These consist of the eastern cities, southwestern centers, and the West Coast. By March distance from Philadelphia meant less than the urban pools of susceptibles in the West, and by April the epidemic had waned.

The severity of the influenza problem in the spring cannot be understated. Figure 7.4 shows the magnitude of the problem in the East. The actual number of cases reported within selected cities during the spring of 1976 are compared with influenza deaths for the winter of 1968–69, when the H3N2 pandemic was officially recognized. The deaths that winter were caused by the entry of a new strain into the country, but those during the spring of 1976 are presumed to have been caused by the prevailing type of influenza that had drifted genetically but not shifted to another type.

Figures 7.5 and 7.6 show a similar pattern for central and western cities. The epidemic in the spring of 1976 was shorter in duration than that of the winter of 1968–69, but in many places it was more intense. National publicity about the possibility of a swine flu epidemic overshadowed an unexpected spring epidemic of H3N2, but to

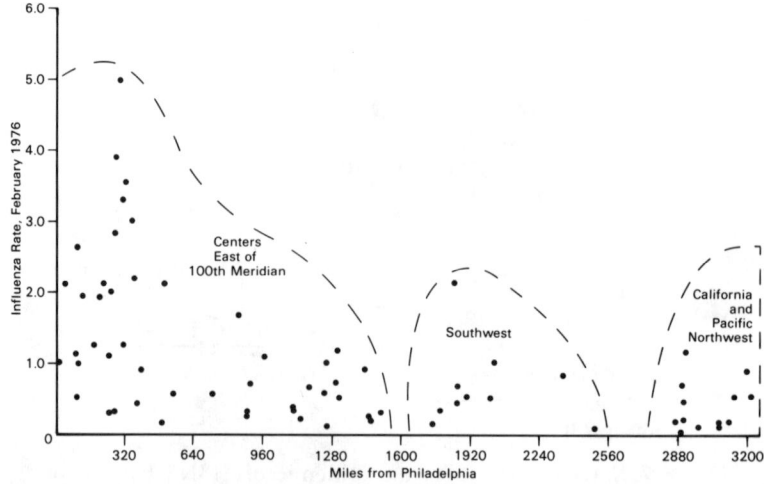

Figure 7.3. Three major regional diffusion patterns could be identified in early 1976.

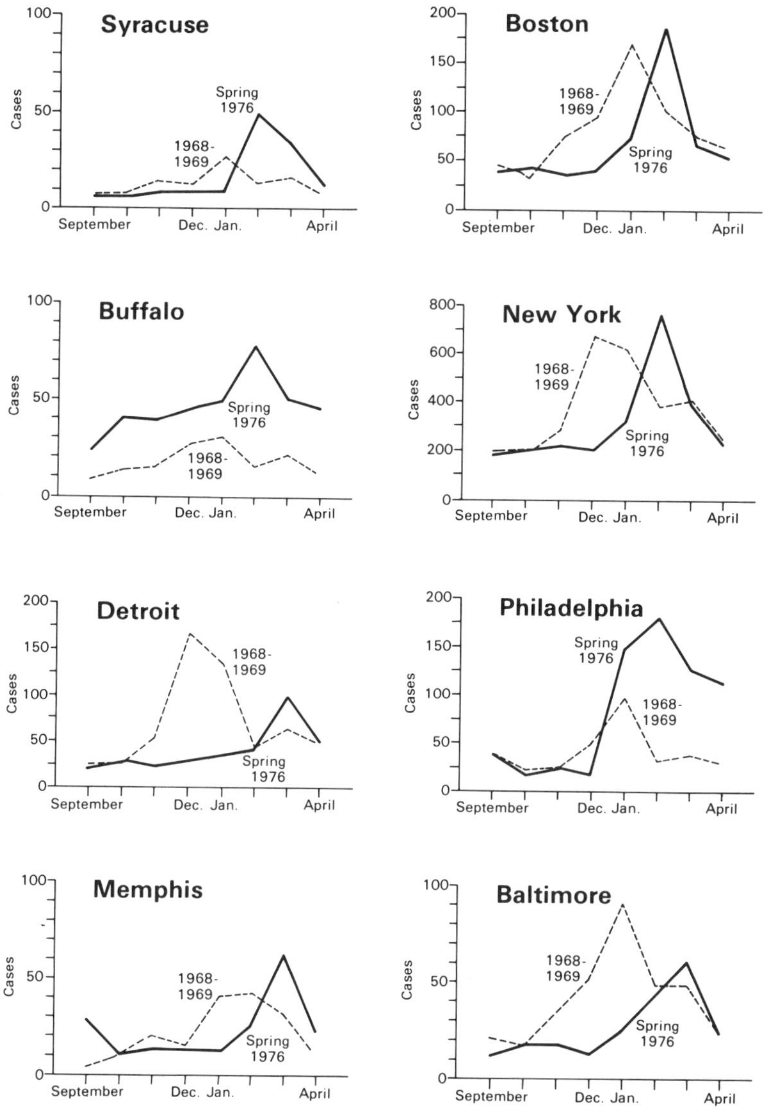

Figure 7.4. These comparisons of outbreaks of influenza, presumed to have been caused by the same strain of virus, show how there were actually more deaths attributed to the disease in the East during the spring of 1976 than the winter of 1968–69.

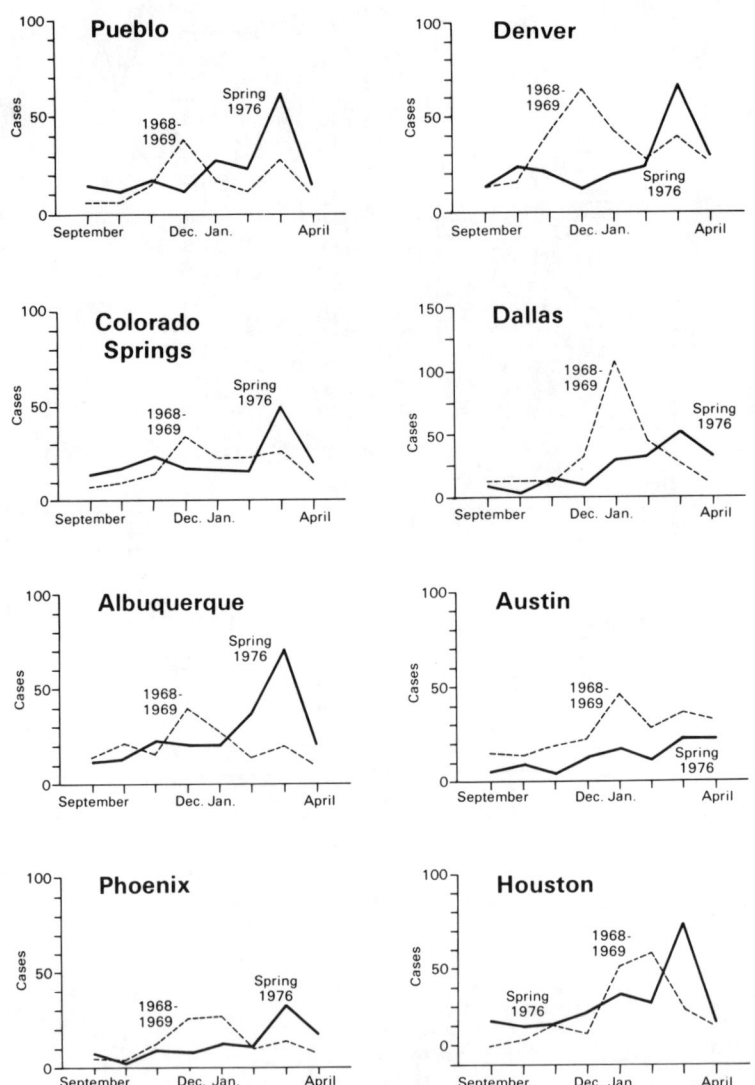

Figure 7.5. Comparisons of H3N2 outbreaks in selected interior cities.

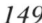

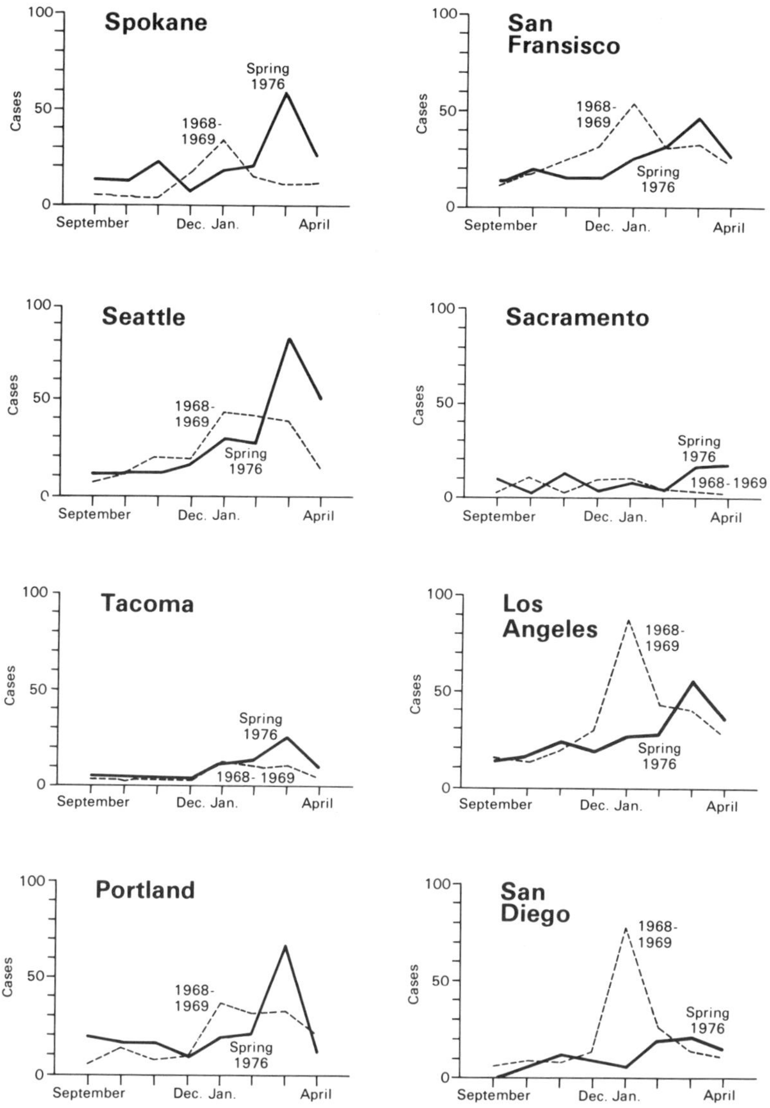

Figure 7.6. With the exception of the Pacific Northwest, the 1976 outbreak of H3N2 seems to have been less severe in the West.

many epidemiologists the increased influenza activity in 1976 suggested the possibility of a herald wave of a possible pandemic during
the winter of 1976–77. A similar sequence of events had unfolded in
1957,[13] and these conditions strengthened the arguments of proponents of a national inoculation program.

The Inoculation Program

In spite of the identification of swine flu in Fort Dix victims and the
spring epidemic, the proposal for a national inoculation program had
lost momentum by April and May. Congressional opposition, presumably because of lagging immunization rates for certain childhood
diseases,[14] seemed to gain sufficient momentum to nullify any proposal for an influenza prevention program. In addition, drug company representatives continued to emphasize the lack of indemnifica-
tion during such a national inoculation program. In fact, there is not
nearly so much profit in influenza vaccine as there is some more
exotic kinds of medication. In spite of these pressures, President
Ford, who supported the program, signed a special appropriations
bill into law (P.L. 94–266) on April 15. In early May, manufacturers of
swine flu vaccine received notice from casualty insurers that their
liability coverage had been canceled, and the production of swine flu
vaccine was brought to a halt.

The CDC continued to press for the program, but support had
waned. Then, it was announced at the beginning of June that one
drug company had used the wrong virus to manufacture two million
doses of vaccine.[15] Epidemiologists from the CDC continued in early
July to search for outbreaks of swine flu elsewhere in the world, but
no cases could be substantiated. However, the outbreak of what later
became known as Legionnaire's Disease during the summer of 1976
may have added the necessary momentum to win public support for
an influenza inoculation program.[16]

During the summer the Public Health Service engaged opinion-
research corporations to determine public attitudes toward inoculation programs, and on August 6, President Ford continued to press
publicly for a national program. Actually, the President stated on July
19 that he would find a way to carry out the immunization program
"with or without the support of Congress." The initial goal of the
Public Health Service was to inoculate approximately 60 percent of
the civilian population above the age of five. Subsequent studies
indicated that inoculating the population over age eighteen would be
sufficient, since the more youthful population was at less risk. In early
August the CDC conducted a poll to determine public demand for

the vaccine and awareness of the potential swine flu problem.[17] At that time, 53 percent of those interviewed said they would obtain a swine influenza shot. Slightly more men than women said they probably would get a vaccination. This was in contrast to 93 percent of those interviewed who said they were aware of the influenza program. A Gallup poll verified those results.

It is somewhat unfortunate that the surveys conducted for the Public Health Service did not identify specific regions of the country, but rather referred only to the West, East, Midwest, and South. Still, slight differences in opinions appeared, and there was a general impression that people in the South were somewhat less informed of the program and slightly less inclined to obtain a vaccination. There was also the contention that no difference existed in percentages of affirmative responses between those residing in cities, suburbs, towns, or rural areas. However, while 94 percent of whites surveyed said they would obtain an inoculation, only 85 percent of blacks responded favorably. As was also expected, higher-income persons said they would probably obtain a vaccination, as did those with at least a college education. The interviews were repeated in September, October, and November. In September the proportion of those indicating they would obtain a swine flu inoculation had changed very little from August. By October the proportion had increased to 57 percent.[18] When asked where they might go to obtain a swine flu shot, about half of those interviewed said they did not know.

The inoculation program began officially in October. The program did not get off to a good start; on October 11, three elderly persons in Pittsburgh died immediately after receiving an inoculation at the same clinic. By mid-October thirty-three persons had died following vaccination, but on October 14, President Ford and his family appeared before television cameras and were given inoculations. Meanwhile, there was little media support for the program, and some newspapers tended to be sensationalistic in swine flu articles.[19] Matters had become even more complicated by mid-November, when the first case of the rare but serious paralytic Guillain-Barré Syndrome associated with a swine flu inoculation was reported. Within a week, however, Missouri public-health officials confirmed a human swine flu case, and increased numbers of people throughout the country lined up for inoculations.[20]

At some juncture during the planning of the inoculation program, health-policy decision makers decided to offer both a monovalent vaccine for swine flu and a bivalent vaccine intended also to induce immunities to H3N2 influenza. This decision is understandable given the nature of the spring 1976 outbreak. Both types of vaccine continued to be administered into December, but problems continued.

Additional cases of Guillain-Barré Syndrome appeared following influenza inoculation, and the program was suspended for one month to allow for an investigation of the strength of the linkage between that ailment and receipt of inoculations. An outbreak of influenza in Miami in January 1977 resulted in a limited continuation of the inoculation program, but in February the Justice Department announced that more than a hundred damage claims totaling more than $11 million had been filed against the federal government under Public Law 94–380.

A change in administration resulted in a new Secretary of Health, Education and Welfare. In February 1976 the director of the CDC resigned. In addition, the inoculation program was permanently halted.[21] These actions were followed by a flood of public criticism of the program, and many opponents from the scientific community reiterated their initial misgivings. While subsequent events, discussed later, may have vindicated many of the more vigorous proponents of the program, the operation sheds some light on the capabilities of the United States health-care delivery system to handle related national emergencies.

Spatial Perspectives on Inoculation Acceptance

The structure of the Public Health Service is such that while national inoculation programs may be initiated at the federal level, individual states implement the vaccination procedures. During the swine flu inoculation program, states were also expected to pay a small portion of the total costs involved. Not all state health departments or their equivalents were enthusiastic about the program for medical as well as cost considerations, so the program was not energetically promoted throughout the country. Also, some state public health officials felt that the program should be administered by the private sector. Conversely, the public's attitude toward the program was not necessarily in consonance with public health decision makers. In spite of differences in opinion regarding vaccine acceptance, an initial examination of state-level proportions of the susceptible populations inoculated suggests strong regional differences.

Figures 7.7 and 7.8, developed from Public Health Service and 1980 census data, attempt to determine if regional differences in vaccine acceptance were apparent for the duration of the program.[22] The four maps show the percentages of the various state populations over the age of eighteen inoculated for the four-month period beginning in October. The overall progression of acceptance gives an impression of more success in the Upper Midwest and Rocky Mountain states than in the Northeast and South or on the West Coast. The cumulative acceptance pattern also seems to confirm some of the findings of the surveys taken prior to the program. Some writers using the same data understandably criticized specific state agencies for not pursuing a more aggressive course of action,[23] and one state governor appeared on television advocating against inoculation.[24]

The four maps in Figures 7.7 and 7.8 also lead to the conclusion that the states with higher rates of acceptance are not heavily populated. Taking the actual number of inoculations as the dependent variable in a least-squares regression with the number of susceptibles as the independent variable results in a strong fit accounting for more than 85 percent of the variance ($r = .933$) (see Fig. 7.9). Many of the states with the highest proportion of inoculations also had the highest positive residuals; states with fewer-than-expected vaccinations included Arkansas, Louisiana, Texas, and South Carolina, as shown in Figures 7.7 and 7.8. Conversely, the results of the regression indicate that the program was far more successful than measures of proportions of acceptance indicate because the actual number of responses was a function of population in spite of variable state policies and procedures.

Yet another policy consideration with inoculation programs in general is that while states have jurisdiction over such matters as dissemination, the national surveillance system is based on reporting cities. The CDC currently relies on reports of influenza deaths from 121 cities, but statistical testing indicates that only 95 cities have been truly reliable during the past fifteen years. It is further possible to extract county-level inoculation counts from the same data base used for the state analysis and isolate 87 of the urban counties in the surveillance system.

Before examining specific urban-acceptance patterns, it is first useful to examine overall county-level trends during the course of the program (Figs. 7.10–7.13). As expected, some counties with the highest proportions of acceptance are located in states with similar patterns. But in many states the high-proportion counties are not the most urbanized. Exceptions include Minnesota and Massachusetts. In some states predominately rural counties registered high rates of acceptance, but more suburbanized counties, usually with higher-income inhabitants, demonstrated higher levels.

Viewing the 87 urbanized counties where a match with effective influenza surveillance systems is obtained, there is a statistically significant relationship between inoculations administered and susceptible populations. Clearly, it is not so strong as the fit with state information, but 45 percent of the variance can be accounted for when numbers of vaccinations are regressed against the susceptible popula-

Percentage of Population Over 18 Years Old
Inoculated by Public Agencies

Through October 1976

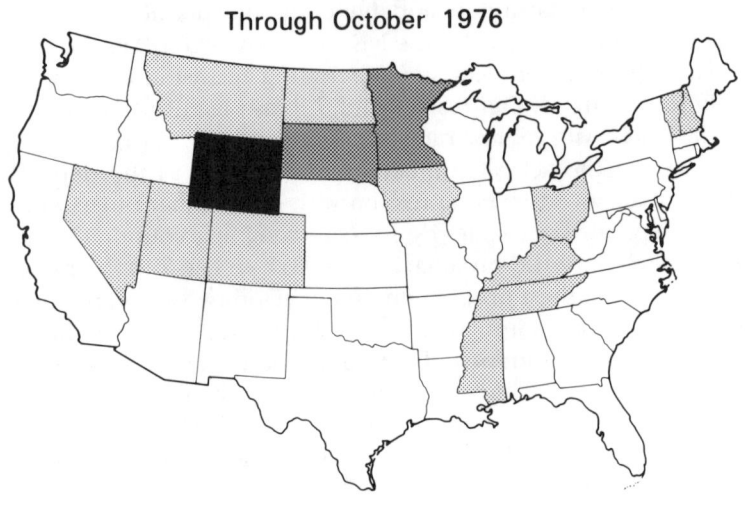

Through November 1976

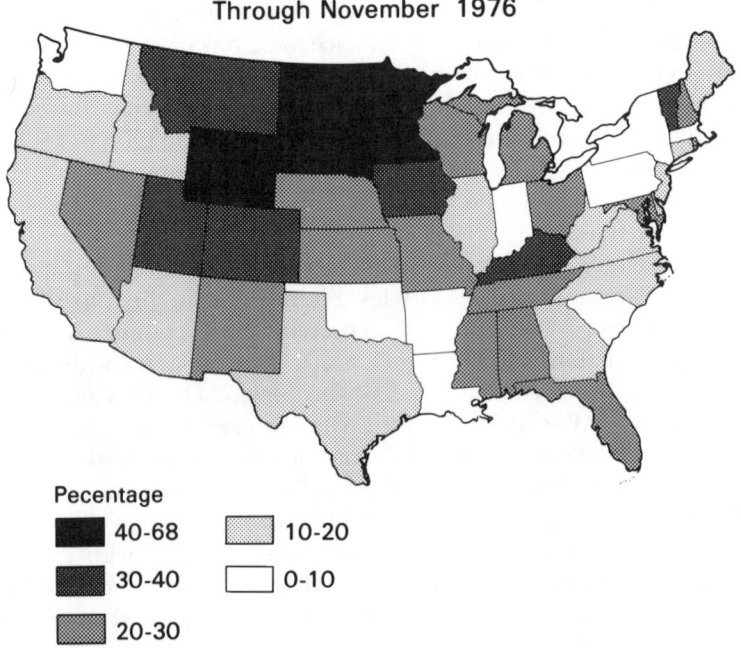

Pecentage

- 40-68
- 30-40
- 20-30
- 10-20
- 0-10

Figure 7.7. The diffusion of "swine flu" vaccine acceptance, using proportions of state adult populations inoculated during October and November 1976.

Percentage of Population Over 18 Years Old
Inoculated by Public Agencies

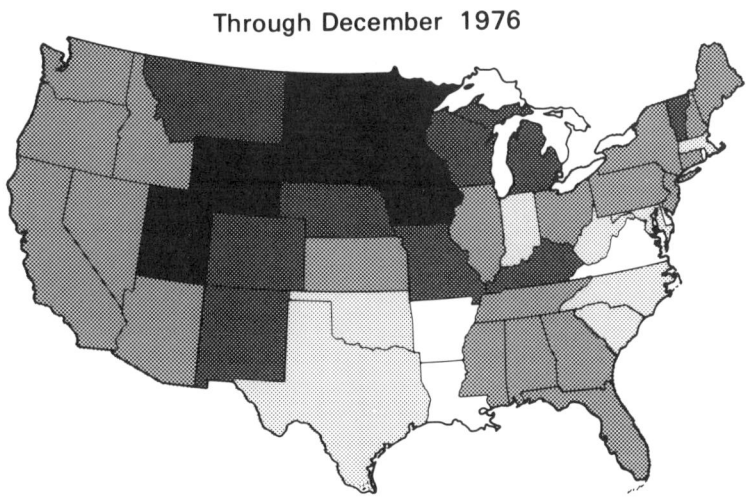

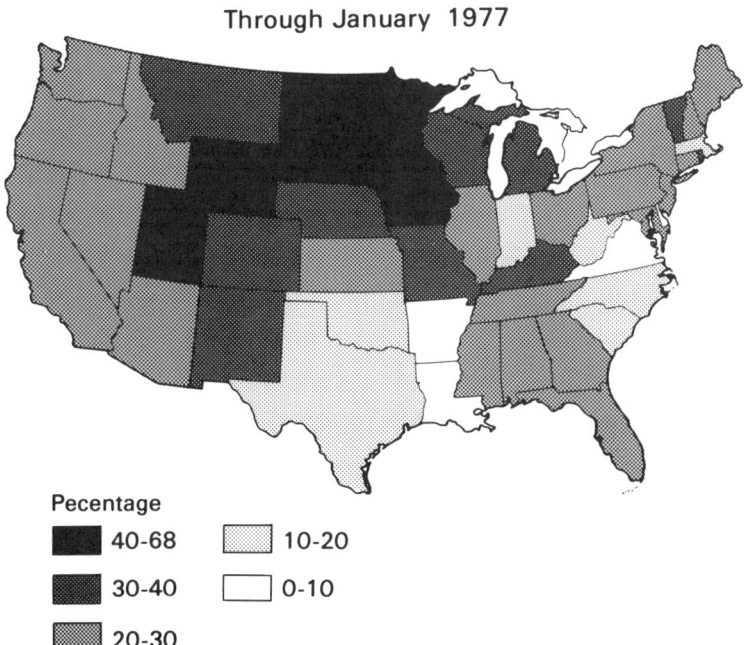

Pecentage

- 40-68
- 30-40
- 20-30
- 10-20
- 0-10

Figure 7.8. The continued diffusion of inoculation acceptance during the national inoculation program.

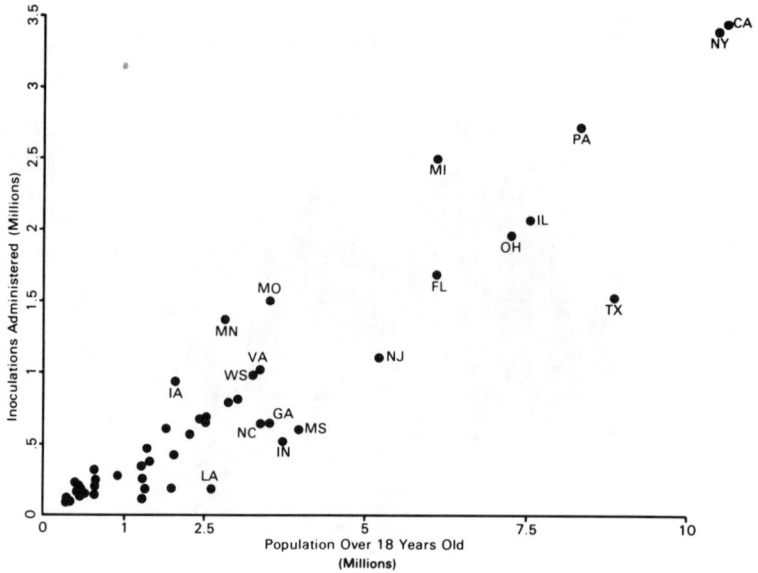

Figure 7.9. Numbers of inoculations administered by public agencies in relation to adult populations.

tions (r = .676). The acceptance trend is also systematically hierarchical. For example, Figure 7.14 depicts the urban-county size-ordering when log ranks of the vaccinations administered are plotted against the numbers of susceptibles. Two urban counties that fall far short of this relationship are those containing Phoenix and Las Vegas.

Chicago, New York, and Los Angeles do not correspond exactly to their actual rank-size position for several reasons. The New York City data were based on boroughs, and the information for Chicago and Los Angeles is county-based. The lower numbers of vaccinations in the Los Angeles area could also have been due to relatively lower numbers of influenza deaths during the spring of 1976 (Fig. 7.5). The high numbers of vaccine recipients in the Chicago area might be attributed to the fact that Chicago was one of the hardest-hit urban centers during the 1918–19 pandemic. In October 1918 approximately 6,000 deaths in Chicago resulted from influenza.[25] The New York City situation is more difficult to analyze because of its complexity, but a 20 percent acceptance rate is probably fairly accurate if one believes the survey findings regarding minority attitudes toward inoculation acceptance.

There is little doubt that the program was a qualified success with regard to the number of persons inoculated. The findings here indicate a systematic response on the part of many in spite of variable

CUMULATIVE PERCENT OF POPULATION
OVER 18 INOCULATED
(Through October 1976)

Percent Inoculated

40-68
30-40
20-30
10-20
1-10
0

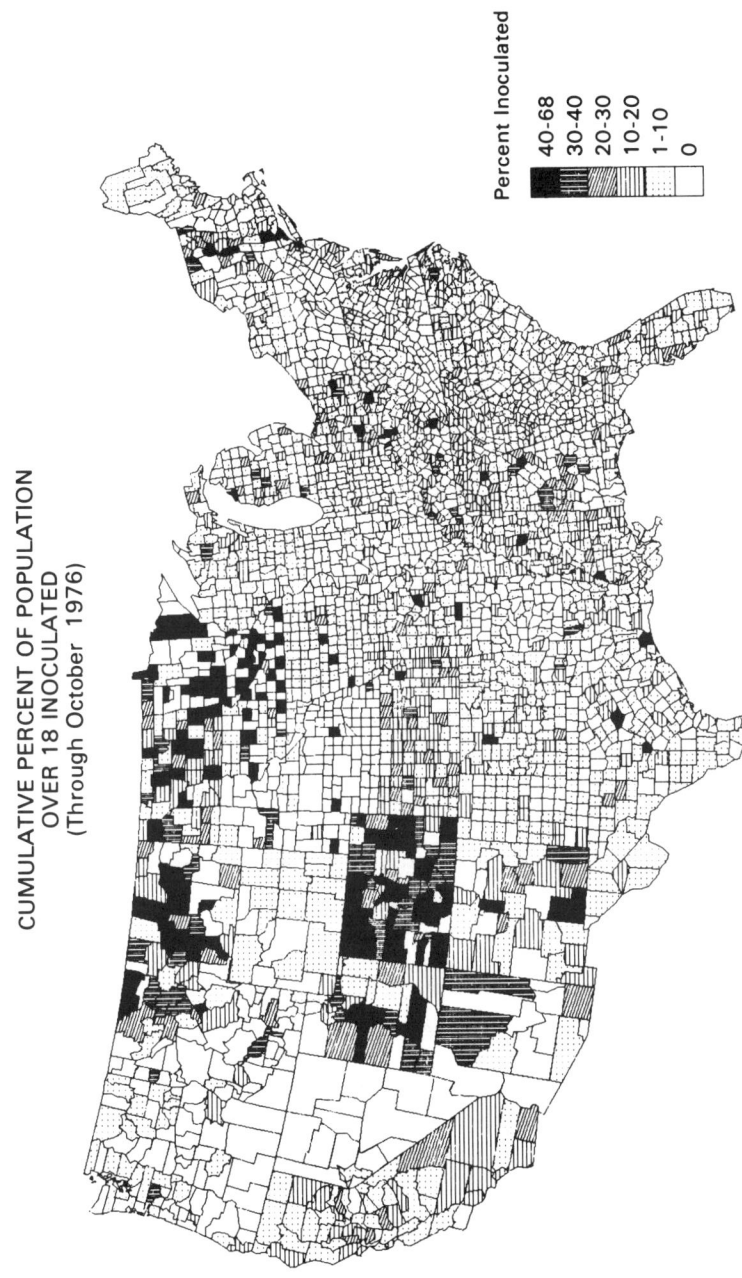

Figure 7.10. Public inoculations administered in counties during October 1976. (Pennsylvania data are incomplete.)

CUMULATIVE PERCENT OF POPULATION
OVER 18 INOCULATED
(October and November 1976)

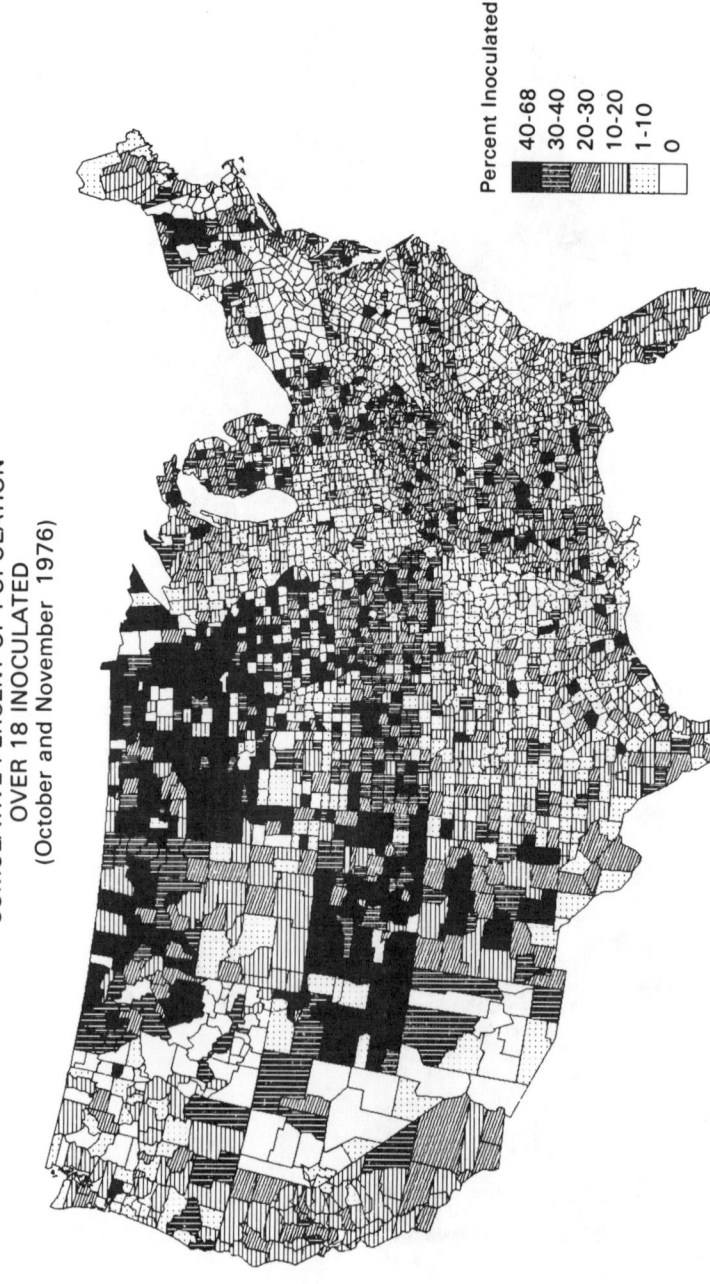

Percent Inoculated

40-68
30-40
20-30
10-20
1-10
0

Figure 7.11. Cumulative county public inoculations by November 1976.
(Pennsylvania data are incomplete.)

CUMULATIVE PERCENT OF POPULATION
OVER 18 INOCULATED
(October through December 1976)

Percent Inoculated

40-68
30-40
20-30
10-20
1-10
0

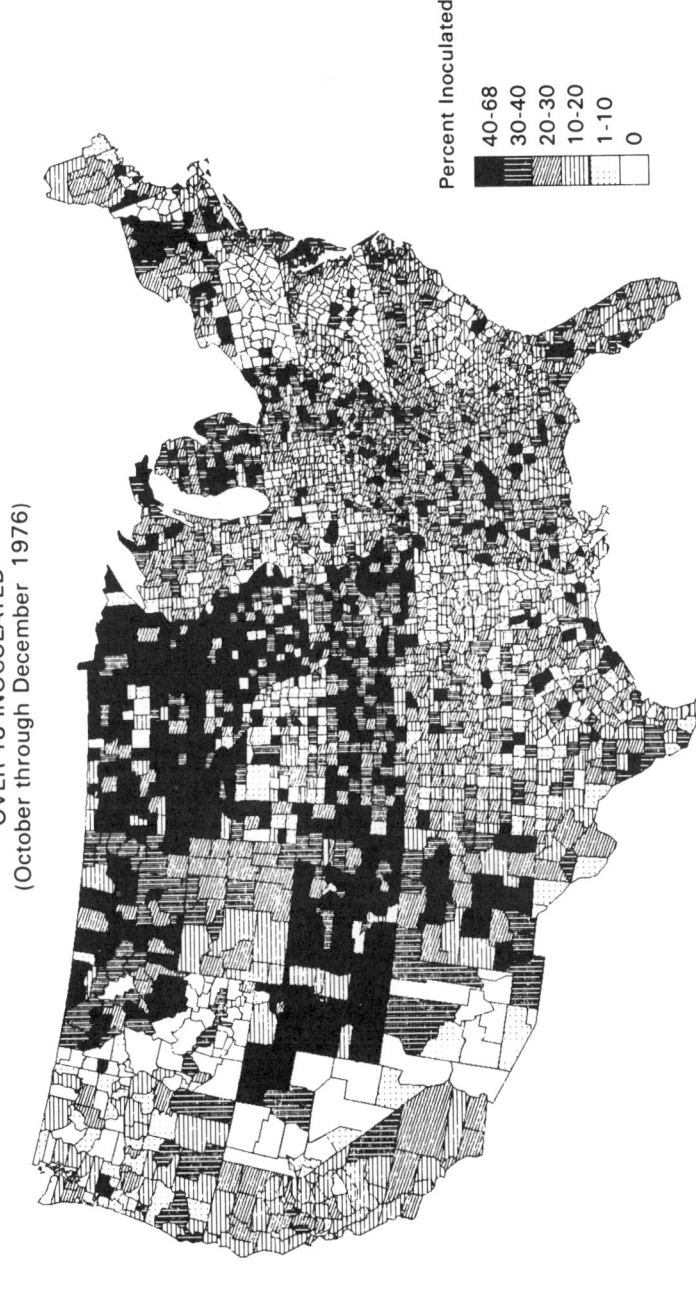

Figure 7.12. Cumulative county public inoculations by December 1976. (Pennsylvania data are incomplete.)

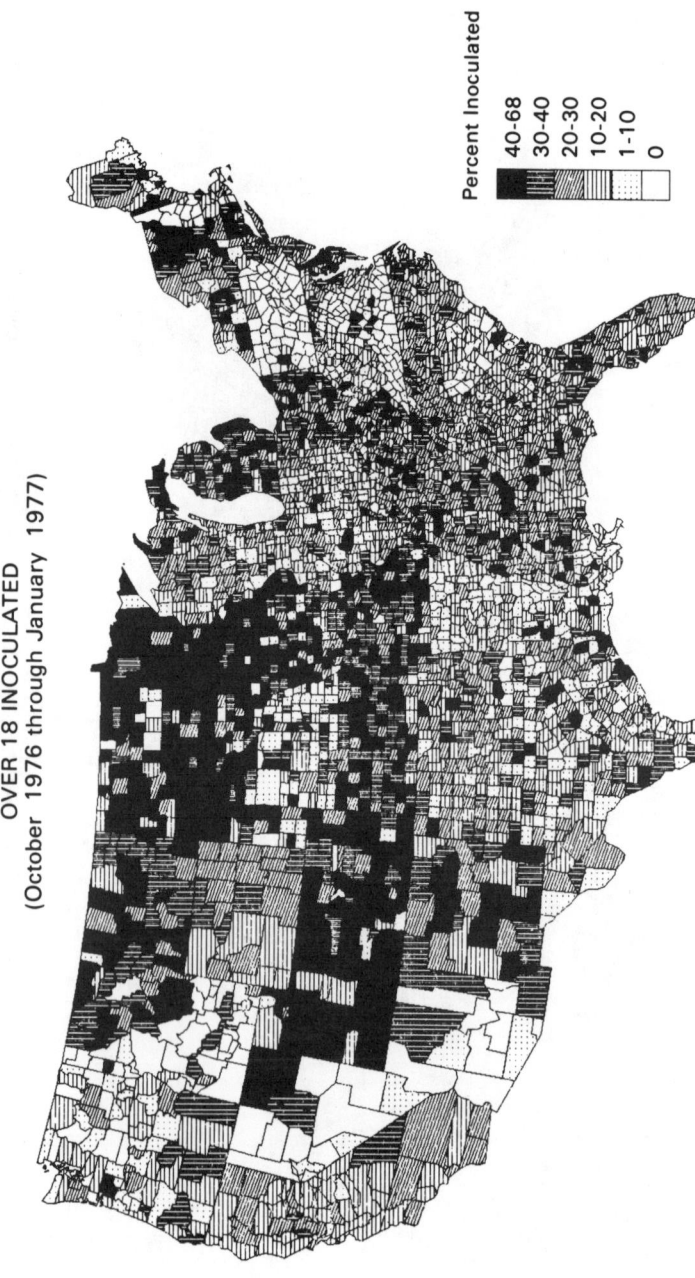

Figure 7.13. Saturation-level vaccine acceptance by the end of the inoculation program. (Pennsylvania data are incomplete.)

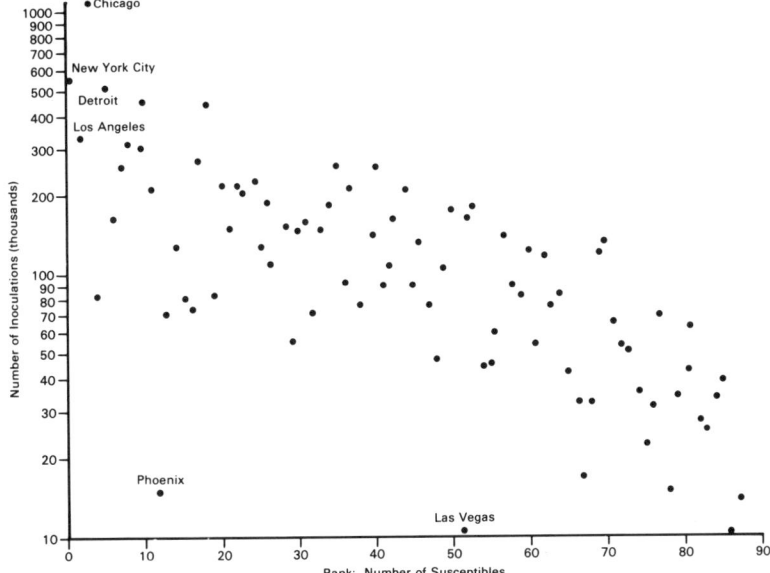

Figure 7.14. Total numbers of inoculated persons in central counties containing CDC influenza-surveillance centers in relation to the number of susceptibles. Clearly, the relationship was hierarchical.

state policies. Had more actual cases of swine flu in humans been discovered during the first nine months of 1976, responses would have been considerably higher. Furthermore, the notice that a new strain of influenza might emerge proved to be substantiated, because that is exactly what happened.

The Aftermath of the Inoculation Program

There was no indication of the appearance of yet another strain of influenza immediately after the inoculation program was curtailed. In fact, during the winter of 1976–77, mortality from influenza was lower than it had been for several years.[26] Public awareness convinced many people to participate in the inoculation program. For comparison, annual mortality trends before, during, and after the program (Fig. 7.12) clearly show the impact of the effort. However, something contrary to assumptions of success also is noticeable in Figure 7.15. Influenza-mortality rates were unexpectedly above the epidemic level during the winter of 1977–78. This condition seemed somewhat paradoxical because more than forty million persons had been inoculated the previous winter. The answer to this puzzle is that they were

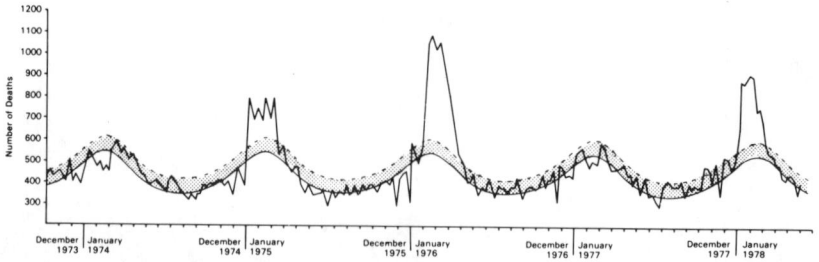

Figure 7.15. The inoculation program was a qualified success, but an epidemic took place during the winter after the program. A different virus was involved.

not inoculated with a vaccine intended to prevent the "new" strain of influenza that emerged in 1977. The type of influenza that surfaced (H1N1) was nearly identical to the strain that caused the epidemic of 1947–48 in many parts of the world. Also with apparent xenogenic origins, the agent has become known as "Russian flu."[27]

Post-Program Influenza Diffusion Patterns

The resurgence of elevated mortality reporting during the winter of 1977–78 was not expected. First and foremost, there was a great deal of relief that a swine flu epidemic never happened. Conversely, following the expectation of some influenza epidemiologists, a new strain, different from that which had prevailed for nearly a decade, did emerge. The strain had apparent beginnings in May 1977 in the People's Republic of China.[28] It spread slowly to reach the Soviet Union and Hong Kong by November and December of that year. Isolates identified within the Soviet Union belonged to the H1N1 type, and the age groups mostly affected there and in other parts of Europe and Asia were young adults and school children. The strain spread through the rest of Europe and the Northern Hemisphere during the winter of 1977–78, and it had reached parts of the Southern Hemisphere by March and April 1979. The virus is considered "historic" because it was the dominant strain from 1947 to 1957, thus explaining the preponderance of youthful morbidity. Mortality was low compared to similar episodes, but influenza deaths in the United States still reached epidemic proportions because the prevailing H3N2 strain continued to cocirculate with the type that reappeared. That condition was the first recorded instance of the failure of a formerly pandemic strain to be supplanted by an emerging viral type.[29]

Together, these strains created the epidemic diffusion patterns in Figures 7.16 and 7.17. The circle sizes on these maps indicate a numerical range of cases (mortality), and during infusion stages, various reporting cities were entered into the diffusion network after reporting in the autumn increased following a summer lull. The shaded circles indicate that the epidemic threshold (more than 4.5 percent of all deaths during the period attributed to influenza) was passed, and the solid circles show when reporting peaked for the season. Regardless of the cocirculation of two viral types, epicenters had formed in the Philadelphia area, Pittsburgh, and upper New York State by September 1977. A negative exponential regression fit with rates (dependent variable) and distance from Philadelphia results in a statistically significant $r = -.549$. The initial epicenters continued to build momentum during October, when the virus in the Chicago area reached epidemic proportions. In addition, reporting was on the increase in several south-central cities. The distance-decay fit for October yielded $r = -.475$, and that statistic had increased to $r = -.551$ by November as the disease continued to spread southward and westward. Epidemic proportions were reached in the Pacific Northwest during December, and reporting also peaked in many places closer to the East Coast. The negative exponential relationship continued to hold up in December with $r = -.528$. By January 1978, when the Public Health Service announced the reappearance of HINI, influenza had peaked in more than half of the major surveillance cities.

The implication is not that influenza epidemiologists were caught unaware. Information about the reappearance of HINI was sent from Moscow to the World Health Organization in December 1977. After influenza surveillance centers around the world were informed, the National Influenza Center in Beijing confirmed that HINI had been detected several months before.[30] Thus, by the time testing could be accomplished in the United States, a fair amount of spatial diffusion had already taken place. The strain of HINI that reappeared was not nearly so virulent as swine flu, and since it had circulated within the population during the 1947–57 period, many people had acquired immunity. Accumulated evidence further suggests that the HINI type also spreads more slowly than the strains that appeared in 1957 and 1968. It is a contention here that while there was cocirculation of both H3N2 and HINI during the 1977–78 season, the latter strain probably did enter the United States in the more urbanized Northeast and slowly diffused to other parts of the country. Such a diffusion pattern can also be explained by the added concentrations of influenza mortality in larger cities, where inoculation acceptance rates were lower.

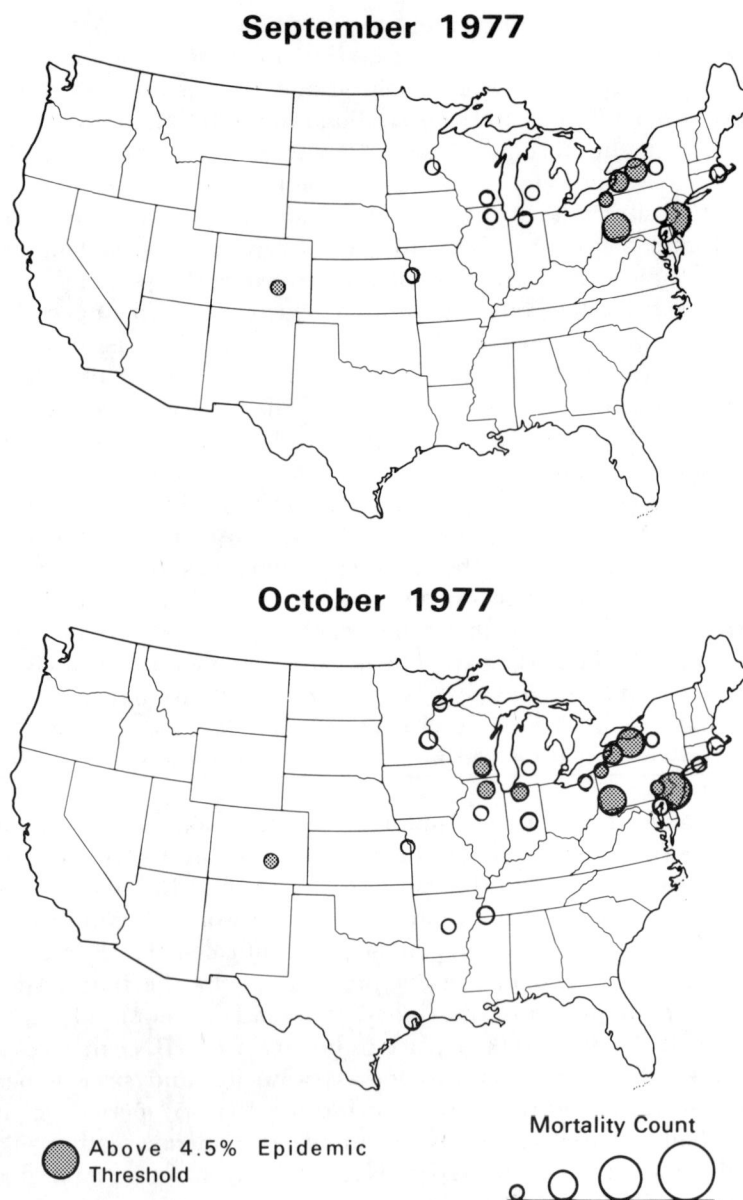

Figure 7.16. These maps show that the 1977–78 influenza epidemic had major origins in the Northeast.

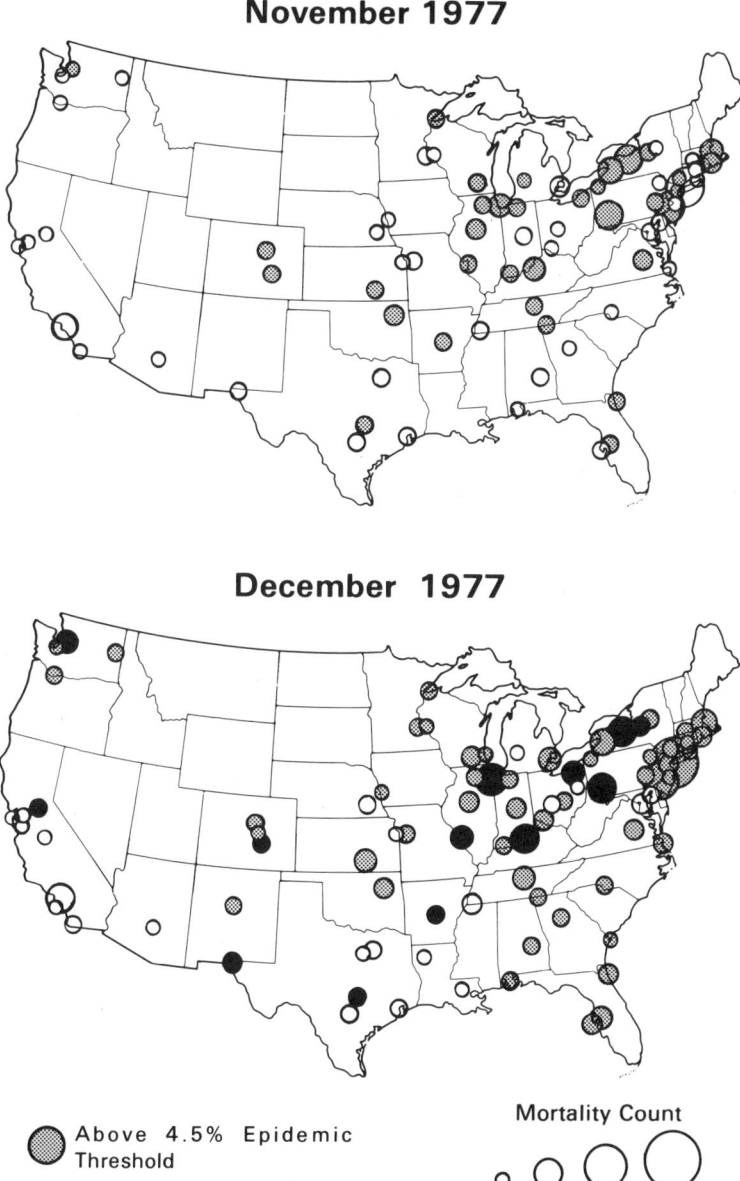

November 1977

December 1977

Above 4.5% Epidemic Threshold

Numerical Peak

Mortality Count

10   75   250   1000

Figure 7.17. The epidemic of 1977 had spread from the Northeast to most other parts of the country by December 1977.

The Importance of Geographical Approaches to Influenza
Diffusion and Inoculation Strategies

The cyclical nature of different strains of influenza emerging or reappearing every decade or so seems to have been reinforced by circumstances in the late 1970s. By the winter influenza season of 1983–84, most influenza isolates were of the HINI type rather than H3N2.[31] Following such logic, there is a good chance that yet another strain of influenza, either known or previously unidentified, will surface during the late 1980s or early 1990s. Influenza is still one of the ten leading causes of death in the United States, and negative attitudes toward prevention programs (including inoculations and other forms of prophylaxis) must be counteracted with positive and timely public-information programs. From a geographical perspective, special emphasis should be placed in large central city areas as well as regions of the country where traditionally conservative attitudes place too much emphasis on the abilities of the private sector to deliver prevention mechansims during such a crisis.

A systematic geographical delivery strategy is also essential for the success of any future influenza-prevention program. This can be accomplished by identifying concentrations of the most susceptible population groups while simultaneously pinpointing those parts of the country that have a higher propensity toward early epicenter formation during an epidemic. Once such areas are identified, estimates of the numbers of possible cases given no prevention procedures can be determined and used as geographical inputs for distribution strategies. Clearly, this cannot be accomplished by using state-level data alone. Instead, units of geographical observation, analysis, and distribution should be based upon our backlog of information pertaining to metropolitan spheres of influence. A systematic hierarchy of national, state, and metropolitan distribution should be more effective than the methods used during the 1976 inoculation program, if such units as the U.S. Department of Commerce–Business Economics Areas are used.[32]

The 1976 program was a qualified success when responses are compared to numbers of susceptibles. Shortcomings included the contagious spread of negative attitudes in already vulnerable locations, lack of support by some state health authorities, insufficient program promotion in many central city areas, the unexpected appearance of rare but serious side effects, and the understandable lack of ability to predict which viral type would actually appear. Anticipation of a swine flu epidemic was not so farfetched, since the HINI strain that emerged is more closely related to swine flu than to the 1957 and 1968 viral types. The relationship between swine flu and the

1977 HINI strain in still distant, however, and the isolation of the latter in the United States in late 1977 does not mean that swine flu was circulating or that it was a precursor strain. The new strain of the early 1980s seems to have followed a well-trodden influenza pathway by emerging in China and spreading to the United States via the Soviet Union. Explanations of why the specific influenza strain that surfaced is a recycled form are more perplexing, as expressed by a recent contribution stating, "It is possible that a 1950 influenza virus was truly frozen in nature or elsewhere and that such a strain was only recently reintroduced into man."[33]

Notes

1. Arthur M. Silverstein, *Pure Politics and Impure Science: The Swine Flu Affair* (Baltimore: The Johns Hopkins University Press, 1981).
2. Stephen C. Schoenbaum, "Influenza Vaccine: Unacceptable or Unaccepted," *American Journal of Public Health* 69 (1979), pp. 219–21.
3. E. O. Kilbourne, "The Influenza Viruses and Influenza: An Introduction," in Edwin O. Kilbourne, ed., *The Influenza Viruses and Influenza* (New York: Academic Press, 1975).
4. Gerald F. Pyle, "Geographical Perspectives on Influenza Diffusion: The United States in the 1940's," in Melinda S. Meade, ed., *Conceptual and Methodological Issues in Medical Geography*, Studies in Geography, no. 15, (Chapel Hill: University of North Carolina, 1980), pp. 222–49.
5. Silverstein, *Pure Politics and Impure Science.*
6. Ibid.
7. Walter Dowdle, "Influenza: Epidemic Patterns and Antigenic Variation," in Philip Selby, ed., *Influenza: Virus, Vaccines, and Strategy* (New York: Academic Press, 1976), pp. 17-21.
8. Martin M. Kaplan and Robert G. Webster, "The Epidemiology of Influenza," *Scientific American* 237 (1977), pp. 88–106.
9. World Health Organization, "A Revised System of Nomenclature for Influenza Viruses," *Bulletin, World Health Organization* 45 (1973), pp. 119–24.
10. Kilbourne, "Influenza Viruses and Influenza."
11. Richard E. Neustadt and Harvey V. Fineberg, *The Swine Flu Affair: Decision-Making on a Slippery Disease* (Washington, D.C. U.S. Department of Health, Education and Welfare, 1978).
12. U.S. Department of Health and Human Services, Public Health Service, Centers for Disease Control, *Influenza Surveillance: Summary,* September 1976–June 1977 (Atlanta: January 1981).
13. Alexander Langmuir, "Asian Influenza in the United States," *Annals of Internal Medicine* 49 (1958), pp. 483–92.
14. Silverstein, *Pure Politics and Impure Science.*
15. Ibid.
16. Gerald F. Pyle, "The MMWR: A Resource for Teaching Medical Geography," *Journal of Geography* 38 (1984), pp. 13–20.
17. Walter J. Gunn, "National Survey of Public Attitudes Towards A/New Jersey/76 Influenza Vaccination: Report No. 1," United States Public Health Service, Center for Disease Control, mimeograph (Atlanta, August 31, 1976).
18. U.S. Department of Health, Education and Welfare, Center for Disease Control, "National Survey of Public Attitudes Towards A/New Jersey/76 Influenza Vaccination: Report No. 3," mimeograph (Atlanta, October 27, 1976).
19. Silverstein, *Pure Politics and Impure Science.*

20. Neustadt and Fineberg, *The Swine Flu Affair.*
21. Ibid.
22. Inoculation count data tape supplied by the Center for Disease Control, Atlanta.
23. Schoenbaum, "Influenza Vaccine."
24. Silverstein, *Pure Politics and Impure Science.*
25. William H. Davis, "The Influenza Epidemic as Shown in the Weekly Health Index," *American Journal of Public Health* 9 (1919), pp. 50–61.
26. U.S. Department of Health and Human Services, *Influenza Surveillance.*
27. M. S. Pereira, "Global Surveillance of Influenza," *British Medical Bulletin* 35 (1979), pp. 9–14.
28. U.S. Department of Health, Education and Welfare, Public Health Service, Center for Disease Control, Atlanta, *Influenza Surveillance*, Report No. 91 (1977).
29. Alan P. Kendal, Gary R. Noble, John J. Skehel and Walter R. Dowdle, "Antigenic Similarity of influenza A (HINI) Viruses from Epidemics in 1977–1978 to "Scandinavian" Strains Isolated in Epidemics of 1950–1951," *Virology* 89 (1978), pp. 632–36; A. P. Kendal, J. Schieble, M. K. Cooney, J. Chin, H. M. Foy, G. R. Noble, "Co-Circulation of Two Influenza A (H3N2) Antigenic Variants Detected by Virus Surveillance in Individual Communities,"*American Journal of Epidemiology* 108 (1978), pp. 308–11; A. P. Kendal, J. M. Joseph, G. Kobayashi, D. Nelson, C. R. Reyes, M. R. Ross, J. L. Sarandria, R. White, D. F. Woodal, G. R. Noble and W. R. Dowdle, "Laboratory-Based Surveillance of Influenza Virus in the United States During the Winter of 1977–78," *American Journal of Epidemiology* 109 (1979), pp. 140–52.
30. Pereira, "Global Surveillance of Influenza."
31. Centers for Disease Control, "Update: Influenza Activity—United States," *Morbidity and Mortality Weekly Report* 33 (1984), pp. 114–15.
32. U. S. Department of Commerce, Social and Economic Statistics Administration, Bureau of Economic Analysis, "Area Economic Projections 1990" (Washington, D.C.: U.S. Government Printing Office, 1979), Stock Number 003–024–00490–9.
33. Katsuhisa Nakajima, Ulrich Desselberger, and Peter Palese, "Recent Human Influenza A(HINI) Viruses Are Closely Related to Strains Isolated in 1950," *Nature* 274 (1978), pp. 334–39; P. Palese and J. F. Young, "Variation of Influenza A, B and C Viruses," *Science* 115 (1982), pp. 1468–75.

8

Simulating Influenza Diffusion

By the mid-1980s the research community was placing proportionately more emphasis on the virology of influenza and less on the epidemiology. Perhaps this increased attention could be attributed to the continuous and seemingly enigmatic phenomenon of cocirculation of H1N1 and H3N2. The fact that H1N1 had not supplanted H3N2 from 1977 to 1985 certainly presented a strong reason for the shift in emphasis.[1] Increased knowledge of the various viruses, in turn, has led to more laboratory surveillance, particularly during nearly continuous periods of heightened influenza activity. The result has been that only impressions of the epidemiology of influenza during the 1980s have emerged, although they are intertwined with mixed reports of "prevailing" strains. Such is the nature of the cocirculation during the 1980s, and both epidemiological and geographical expositions of influenza trends are strongly influenced by this circumstance. In order to accomplish one of the major purposes of this study—the simulation of possible future diffusion pathways—it is necessary to develop an understanding of epidemiological-virological conditions during the 1980s, as well as geographical determinants of changing influenza patterns.

Endemic and Epidemic Conditions

Studying influenza trends in the 1980s requires close scrutiny of seasonal variations in mortality because, by current definitional standards, almost every winter season from the reintroduction of H1N1 into the U.S. population in 1977 to the winter of 1984–85 can be considered "epidemic." CDC influenza researchers in the 1980s define influenza deaths as a percentage of the total deaths recorded from surveillance cities. The epidemic threshold is exceeded when more than 4.5 percent of all deaths during any given week are attributed to pneumonia-influenza.[2] This procedure is considered a refinement over the actual numbers measure of the Serfling method.

However, one aspect of temporal trends that emerged by using this method was the impression of a continuous stream of epidemics. While this is not surprising because two major strains continued to circulate, it is still necessary to separate significant epidemic conditions from endemic circumstances in the process of modeling spatial-diffusion patterns. Figure 8.1 enables us to make a comparative distinction. Using the ratio method, it is clearly apparent that the two most serious influenza outbreaks occurred during the winters of 1977–78 and 1980–81. In spite of the apparent general trend suggesting increased proportions of influenza deaths, these two winters were, at least by numerical standards, the most epidemic.

Clearly, the cocirculation of two strains is an endemic circumstance, and this can be demonstrated by comparing the geographical patterns of the two most pronounced outbreaks shown in Figure 8.1. The epidemic of 1980–81 was more "unexpected" than that of the 1977–78 winter. During the latter episode, there was advance warning that a "new" strain was circulating in Europe.[3] In addition, there were laboratory confirmations of H1N1 in the United States in early February 1978.[4] Conversely, there were no early reports of a possible epidemic during the autumn of 1980. There were two major reasons for the lack of any major public notification of an epidemic: (1) the epidemic threshold was not exceeded until mid-December,[5] and (2) by then an additional major strain of influenza had emerged. The first reason is most easily understood by examining Figure 8.2. The epidemic threshold was exceeded in December and the actual epidemic peaked in late January 1981. In addition, laboratory surveil-

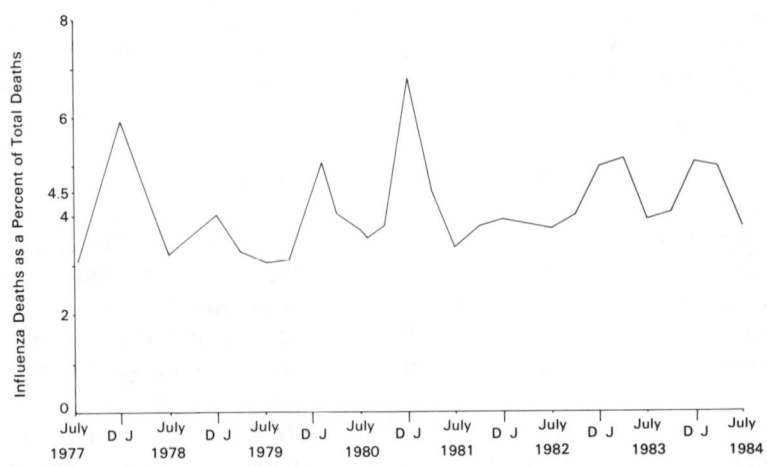

Figure 8.1. Cycles of influenza mortality during the early 1980s expressed as proportion of total deaths.

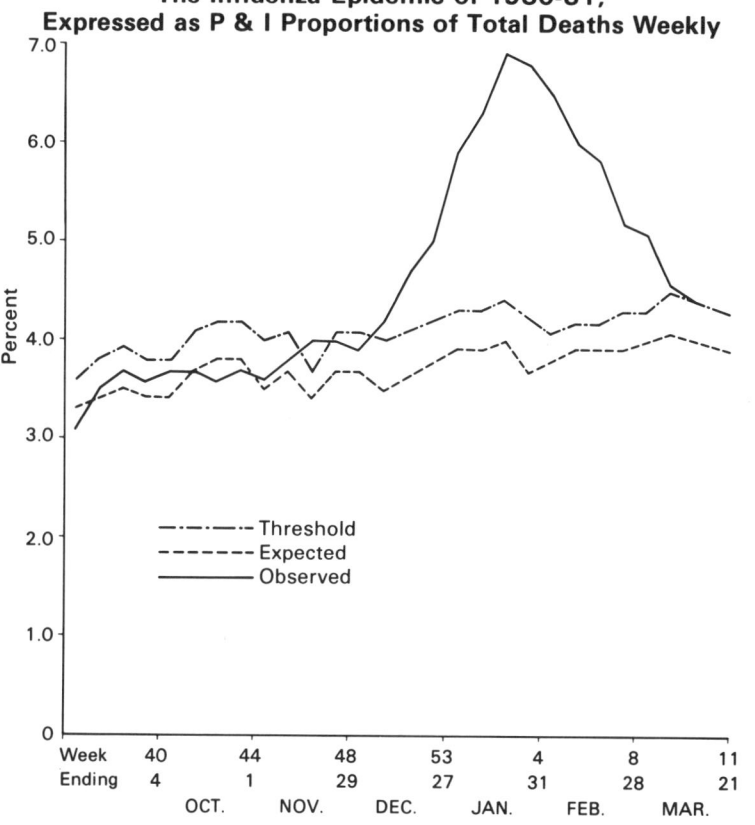

Figure 8.2. The epidemic of 1980–81.

lance for influenza virus infections during that winter had indicated that H3N2 was more pronounced during the earlier part of the season,[6] and isolates of H1N1 gradually increased during January 1981 (Fig. 8.3).

Patterns of spatial diffusion were also different during the two epidemics. For example, the diffusion patterns uncovered in Chapter 7 (Figs. 7.16 and 7.17) indicate that, on the basis of actual mortality counts, influenza generally spread from east to west during the autumn of 1977. The 1980–81 patterns were much more complex. In fact, there was considerable influenza activity below the epidemic threshold level in two outbreaks during the summer and fall of 1980. This sequence of events is depicted in Figures 8.4 to 8.7. As if to suggest summers to come during the early 1980s, cities in widespread locations exceeded the threshold during August 1980. Still, there were insufficient deaths to indicate a national problem. The early-

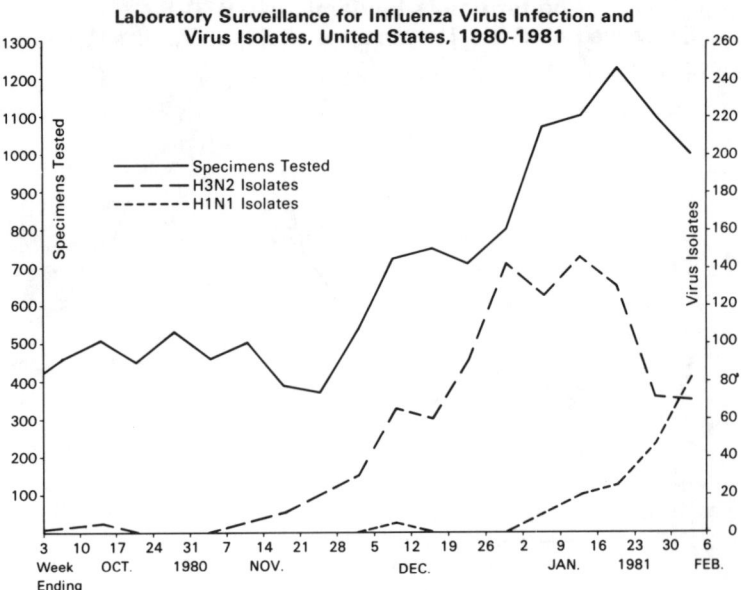

Figure 8.3. Isolations of both H3N2 and H1N1 during the epidemic of 1980–81.

season flare-up increased in September but then declined somewhat in October. While some cities reached peak proportions in December, it was not until January that the national epidemic was fully realized. Influenza deaths declined during February and March 1981.

Summary comparisons of the two epidemics also help us to understand the different spatial-diffusion patterns that result from the introduction of a new strain as opposed to continued circulation of existing strains. As with the summary mapping of the epidemics in the winters of 1918–19 (Chapter 3), 1929–29 (Chapter 3), and 1947–48 (Chapter 4), epidemic waves were identified with harmonic measurements for the 1977–78 and 1980–81 seasons. Figures 8.8 and 8.9 show the different diffusion patterns. The actual methodology, while infrequently used in epidemiology, has been extensively applied in the earth sciences for decades. Paul Schureman's *Manual of Harmonic Analysis and Prediction of Tides* contains an excellent historical statement on the method.[7] Devised by Sir William Thomson in about 1867, the method's underlying principle is that periodic oscillations can be resolved into the sum of a series of harmonic motions. The harmonic relationship between ocean tides and celestial bodies was then determined. During the early 1960s Horn and Bryson[8] and Sabbagh and Bryson applied harmonics to weather data.[9] In such spatial analyses a

Fourier series is fitted to data from different geographical points in a temporal sequence, such as twelve consecutive months. The key elements to be extracted are the amplitude, phase, and variance over several harmonics (six is conventional). One of the most succinct explanations can be found in Brooks and Carruthers,[10] and their computations were used for the harmonic maps produced in this study. Influenza reporting was initially combined from weekly mortality counts into twelve consecutive one-month periods beginning with July of one year and continuing through June of the next. The process is fairly straightforward. Initially, the coefficients A and B are identified, where:

$$A = \frac{\sum_{i=1}^{12} \left(\cos \left(\frac{iH\pi}{6} \right) * OBS_i \right)}{6};$$

for harmonics = 1, 2 . . . , 6

$$B = \frac{\sum_{i=1}^{12} \left(\sin \left(\frac{iH\pi}{6} \right) * OBS_i \right)}{6}$$

The amplitude (AMP) is determined as:

$$AMP = \sqrt{A^2 + B^2}$$

and the normalized amplitude is AMP divided by the mean. The variance (VAR) is determined as:

$$VAR = \begin{cases} \dfrac{(AMP)^2}{2}, & \text{for } H = 1, 2, 3, 4, 5 \\ AMP^2, & \text{for } H = 6 \end{cases}$$

and the phase is determined by:

$$\tan^{-1} \left(\frac{B}{A} \right)$$

Similar procedures were used by Brier in 1966, 1968, and 1978.[11,12]

Mathematically, the results of such measurements are extremely useful for spatial-temporal comparison because many of the minor oscillations are smoothed over. For comparisons of influenza diffusion, the method is additionally useful because it seems to solve the problem so often encountered when large cities have substantial

August 1980

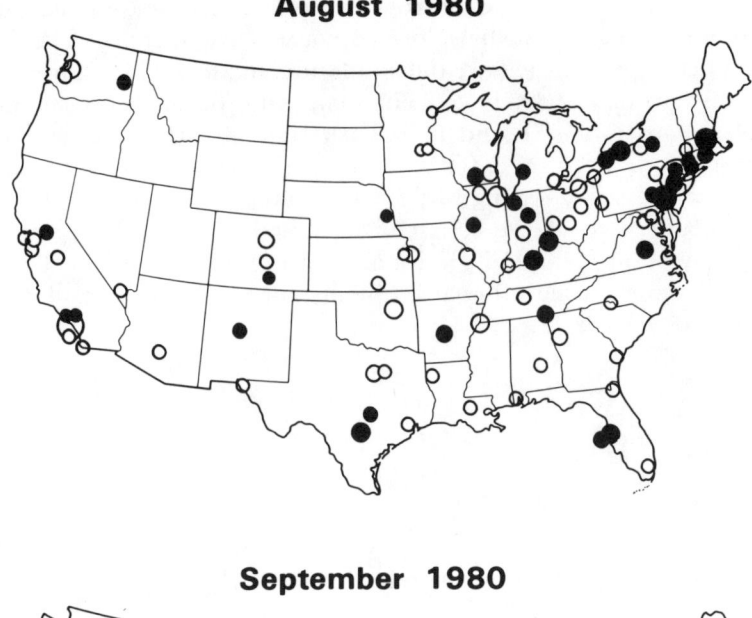

September 1980

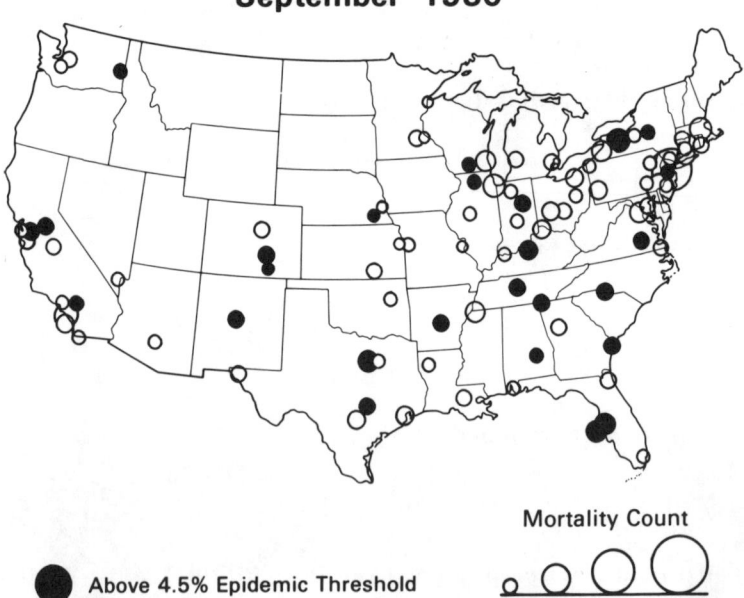

Mortality Count

● Above 4.5% Epidemic Threshold

10   75   250   1000

Figure 8.4. Influenza outbreaks during the late summer and early autumn of 1980. The widespread reporting was due to endemic cocirculation of two strains.

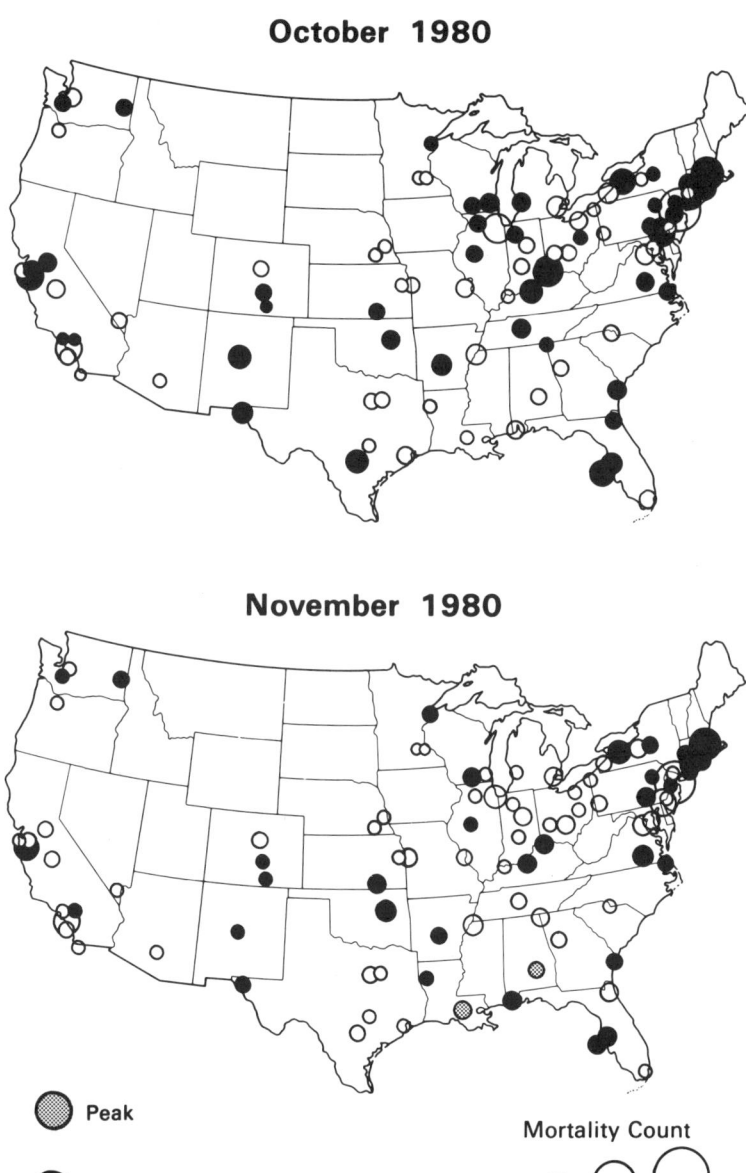

Figure 8.5. Continued cocirculation during the autumn of 1980.

December 1980

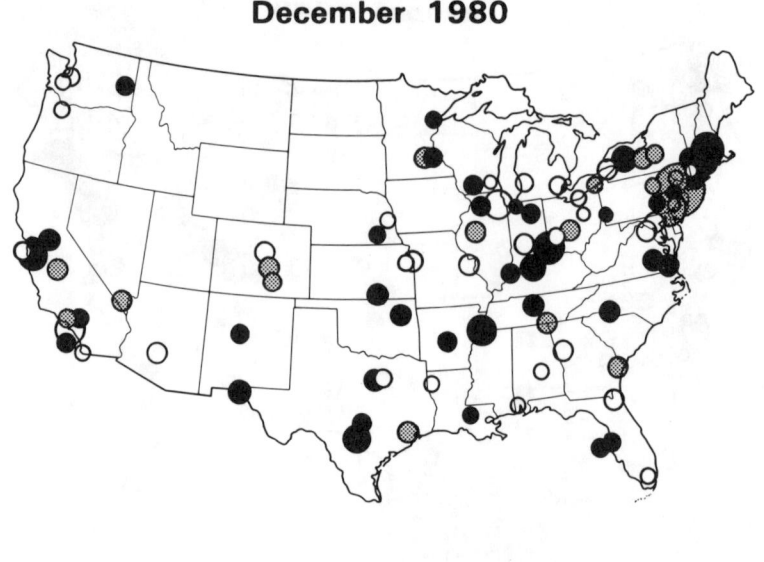

January 1981

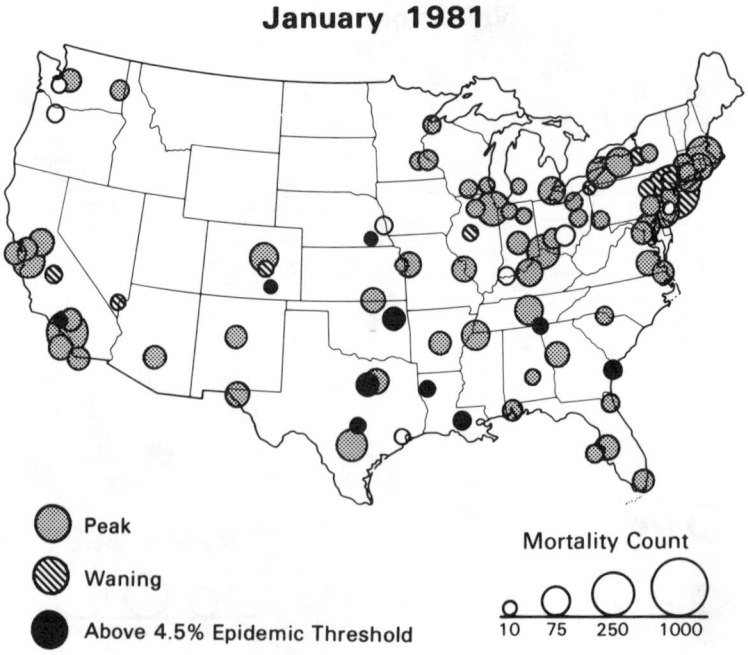

⬤ Peak

◐ Waning

● Above 4.5% Epidemic Threshold

Mortality Count

○ ○ ○ ○
10 75 250 1000

Figure 8.6. By January 1981, influenza mortality had peaked in most parts of the country, and a "surprise" epidemic had been announced.

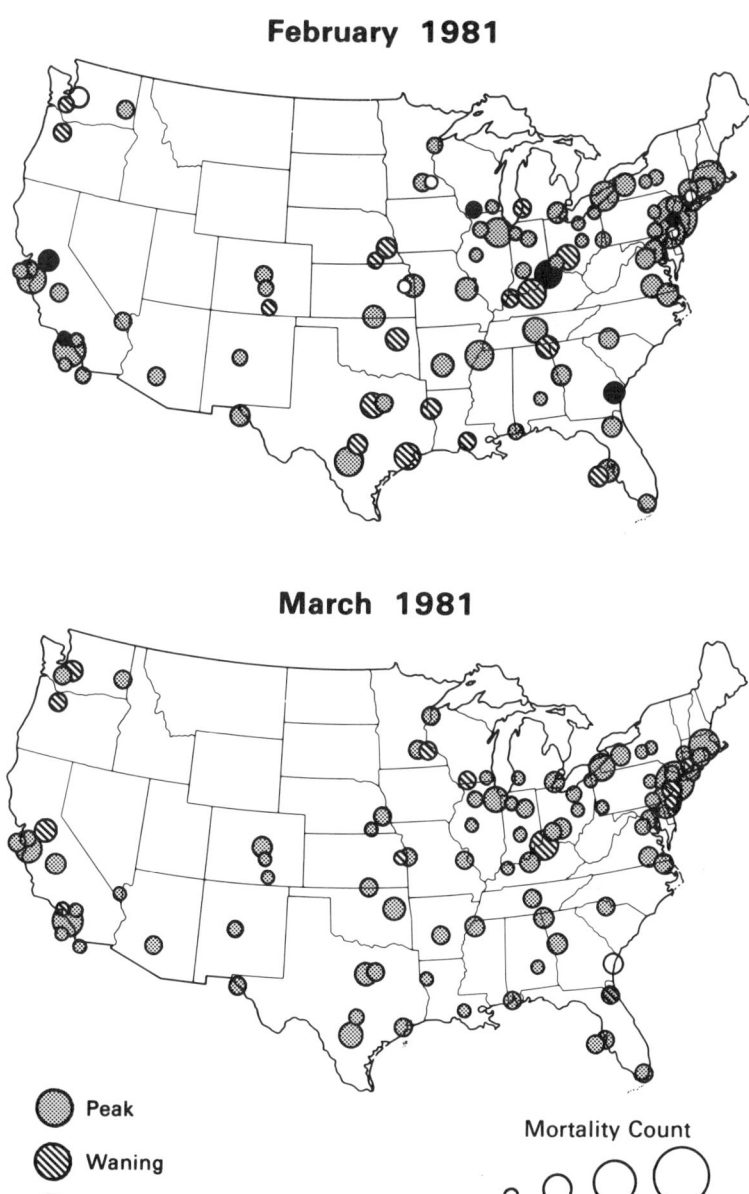

February 1981

March 1981

Peak

Waning

Above 4.5% Epidemic Threshold

Mortality Count

10   75   250   1000

Figure 8.7. Influenza mortality declined during early 1981.

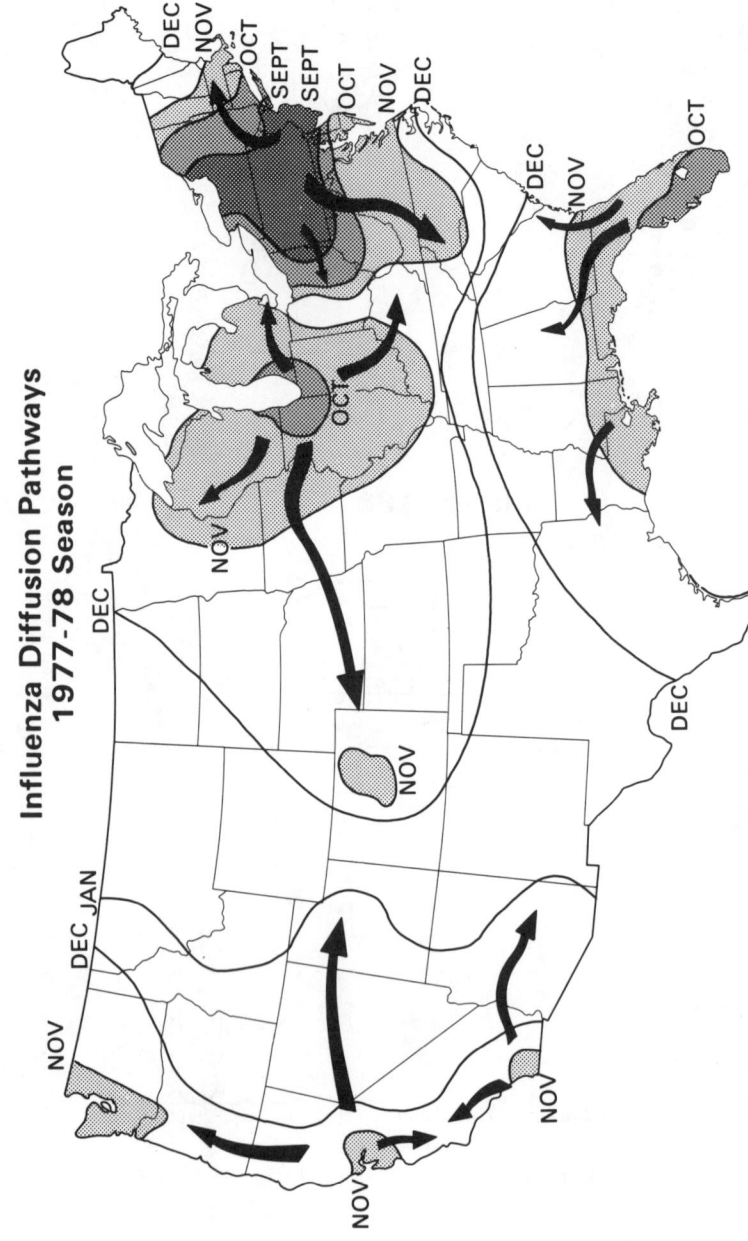

Figure 8.8. Reconstructed influenza diffusion pathways during the autumn of 1977, using harmonic measures.

**Postulated Influenza Pathways:
Autumn of 1980**

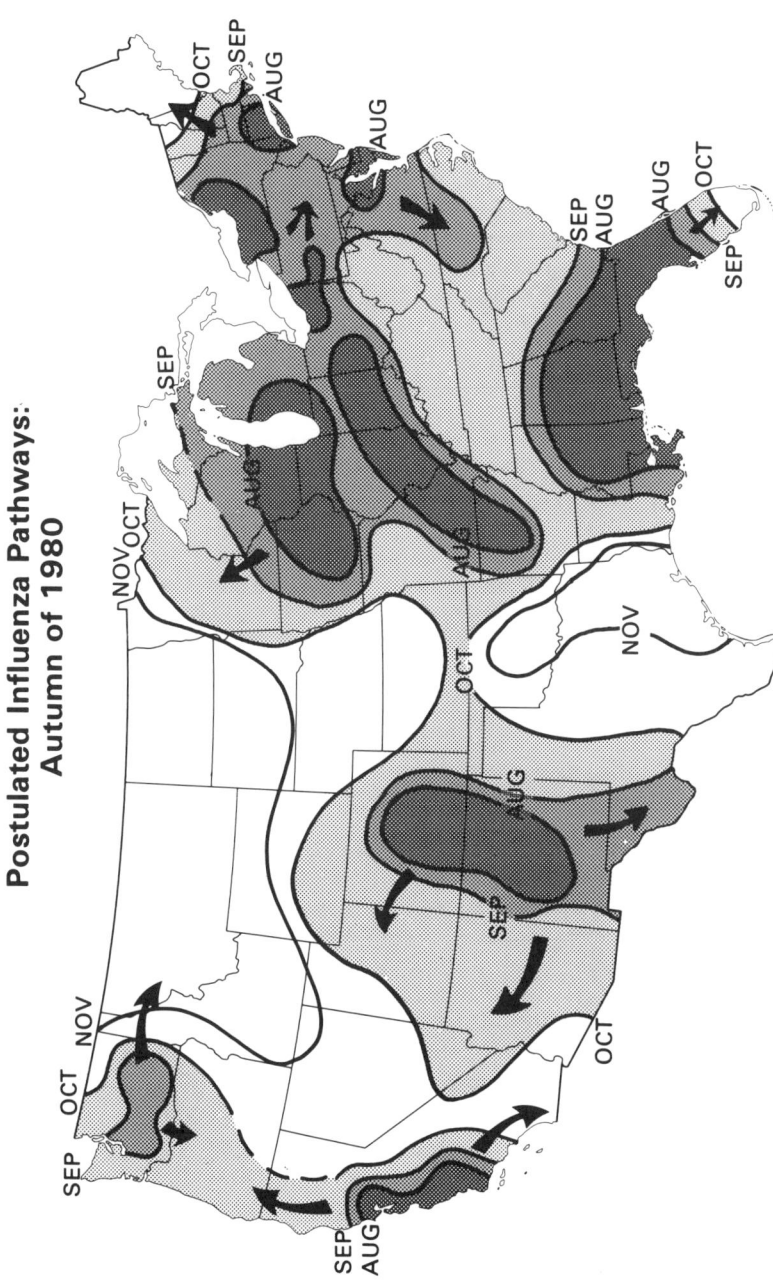

Figure 8.9. Reconstructed diffusion pathways during the autumn of 1980. The multiple-outbreak epicenters indicate endemic influenza.

Table 8.1   Harmonic Calculations for New York City, 1977–78 Season

Deaths per 100,000	
July	354
August	291
September	285
October	380
November	280
December	509
January	647
February	421
March	330
April	394
May	265
June	267

Harmonic	A	B	Amplitude	Normalized	Mean	PHASE Radians	Degrees	Months
1	− 170.53	2.67	107.56	0.29	368.58	3.117	178.58	5.95
2	65.17	0.87	65.17	0.18	368.58	0.007	0.38	0.01
3	− 38.83	21.00	44.15	0.12	368.58	0.882	50.53	1.68
4	75.17	− 19.34	77.62	0.21	368.58	1.508	86.39	2.88
5	− 0.14	11.33	11.33	0.03	368.58	0.317	18.14	0.60
6	− 16.83	0.00	16.83	0.05	368.58	0.524	30.00	1.00

SUMMARY OF VARIANCE FOR ALL HARMONICS

Harmonic	Variance	Percent of Total
1	5784.58	47.250
2	2123.72	17.347
3	974.513	7.960
4	3012.06	24.603
5	64.196	0.524
6	283.361	2.315

numbers of deaths but contain so many people that the rates calculated are not a true reflection of the problem. For example, comparisons of New York City and most other cities usually present such a problem because rates for New York are relatively low, but numbers of deaths are not. Tables 8.1 and 8.2 help explain how the use of the harmonic peak eliminates the problem. Using mortality rates by months, the amplitude, phase, and variance have been calculated for the 1977–78 and 1980–81 influenza seasons. The actual time of peaking is determined by converting the phase angle radians and degrees into months. In order to map the results of harmonic fit for numerous points, a certain amount of temporal "backtracking" as

Table 8.2 Harmonic Calculations for New York City, 1980–81 Season

Deaths per 100,000

July	289
August	195
September	230
October	292
November	299
December	623
January	574
February	354
March	258
April	288
May	244
June	229

						PHASE		
Harmonic	A	B	Amplitude	Normalized	Mean	Radians	Degrees	Months
1	− 134.24	24.15	136.39	0.42	322.92	2.964	169.80	5.66
2	78.00	− 51.67	93.56	0.29	322.92	2.849	163.24	5.44
3	− 33.67	38.50	51.14	0.16	322.92	0.763	43.72	1.46
4	37.83	− 35.80	52.08	0.16	322.92	1.381	79.15	2.64
5	25.40	16.35	30.21	0.09	322.92	0.114	6.55	0.22
6	− 14.50	− 0.00	14.50	0.04	322.92	0.524	30.00	1.00

SUMMARY OF VARIANCE FOR ALL HARMONICS

Harmonic	Variance	Percent of Total
1	9301.11	54.684
2	4377.04	25.734
3	1307.85	7.689
4	1356.35	7.974
5	456.340	2.683
6	210.250	1.236

indicated within Chapter 1 is necessary to develop diffusion maps. The results are encouraging.

The diffusion patterns shown in Figures 8.8 and 8.9 not only assist in the identification of the entry of a new strain (1977), but they also exemplify multiepicenter outbreaks of an *epidemic* of *endemic* influenza (1980–81). Comparisons with previous years also reveal some striking results not previously reported in the influenza literature. Specifically, when the diffusion patterns shown in Figure 8.8 are compared with Figure 4.7 (1947–48) and Figure 3.4 (1918–19), the similarities become incredible. Furthermore, the strain of H1N1 reintroduced in 1977 is extremely close to the 1947 virus. Also, both are presumed to be closely related to the 1918–19 strain. It is also of interest to note that the multiple-epicenter patterns of the 1980–81 season more closely resemble the patterns of the 1928–29 and 1968–68 epidemics than any of the 1970s outbreaks.

In spite of the importance of harmonic techniques in depicting patterns of spread, the measures derived are of limited value in modeling possible future diffusion pathways. One exception to this observation is that harmonic analysis can assist in determining early outbreak epicenters over five-to-six-year periods, and that information can in turn be used in simulation procedures. However, alternative methods with elements common to both of the disciplines of epidemiology and geography are required. In addition, it is also necessary to determine *why* various viruses behave the way they do spatially.

The Search for an Explanation

So far, little integration has been achieved between standard epidemiological techniques and the most successful diffusion models used by geographers. A recent attempt toward such integration can be found in the works of Cliff et al. with measles diffusion modeling in Iceland,[13] but influenza unfortunately does not seem to behave with such mathematical regularity. In addition, the geographical perspective is not a major consideration in the majority of influenza-diffusion models now in use, since they range from family studies to clinics and small communities. Some limited geographical considerations are given to spatial dimensions in the work of Elveback and her colleagues in their development of nonhomogeneous, nonrandom-mix models that assist in understanding the diffusion of H2N2 and H3N2 within communities of up to 1,000 persons.[14] Bailey has supported the contention that it is easier to model measles than influenza diffusion, and he has in addition suggested that problems seem to arise when influenza diffusion is attempted within urban settlements of more than 250,000 persons,[15] a further indication of the "large numbers" problem identified earlier. The more recent efforts in modeling influenza diffusion in the Soviet Union by Baroyan and co-workers attempt to predict geographical-spread pathways for the entire country, but as with the efforts of American epidemiologists, it appears that few, if any, geographers have been included in the Russian modeling applications.[16] The epidemiological literature does contain some general geographical considerations. Fine has recently summarized some of these issues.[17] Historical accounts include notions that influenza at times has the ability to travel rapidly over great distances, and Fine suggests that since humans clearly are large host groups the influenza viruses seem to "go with the people." Some epidemiologists have argued that influenza follows existing transportation routes, while others have stated that the disease seems to spread in a "direct" geographical fashion in spite of the transportation network. Modes of transportation might influence rate of spread but not direction. On a global basis, there does seem to be evidence of "transequatorial swing" depending on which hemisphere is experiencing winter, but this phenomenon is not that regular because major influenza epidemics have started during the summer in Northern Hemisphere locations. For example, H2N2 spread from China into both hemispheres during the summer of 1957. One common element to most epidemiological approaches is the recognition of population concentrations as masses of attraction. While vaguely defined in epidemiological approaches, population potential is well understood in related geographical studies, as is evidenced by the examination of influenza diffusion in England and Wales by Hunter and Young[18] and general studies of spatial diffusion by Brown and his co-workers.[19]

The actual influenza-diffusion models have been developed in the traditional epidemiological contexts of either "family" or "community" studies, and each demonstrates a somewhat different approach. There is much dialogue within the literature on influenza spread about why community models seem to work better than family models, thus the implication of scale differences. Anything above the community level is considered a "large population," and the best definition of community appears to be a size not exceeding 1,000 persons. In spite of tremendous variations in population size from one location to another, essentially the same methods have been used. The models have much in common. For example, they often attempt to consider a chain of transmission that includes:

1. clinical aspects of the disease, particularly the proportion of infections known,
2. the incubation period, or time lag from infection to onset,
3. the duration of infectiousness,
4. mortality, or morbidity when known,
5. period of infectiousness,
6. the latent period from infection to infectiousness, and
7. the pool of susceptible individuals.

A concept that has been given considerable attention in the literature is the notion of "secondary attack rate"—the rate of spread after initial cases in populations have been confirmed. Once again, however, secondary rates that have been established to measure incubation, latent, and infectiousness periods yield a wide range of results.

According to Fine, there are two classical approaches to the modeling problem: "mass action" and "Reed-Frost"-type formulations. The mass-action approach dates to the early twentieth century.[20] Stated in discrete form:

$$C_{t+1} = S_t * C_t * b$$

where C_{t+1} = the number of infected and infectious at time $t+1$
S_t = the number of susceptibles at time t
b = the "transmission coefficient."

The latter term is a parameter that has been given such labels as "transmission rate," "contact rate," "force of infection," and "infection rate" by different authors. Fine suggests "probability of effective contact." Continuous time variants of this model can be expressed:

$$\frac{dy}{dt} = x * y * \beta$$

where y = number of infectious cases
x = number of susceptibles
β = "transmission rate"
$\frac{dy}{dt}$ = derivitive of infectious cases with respect to time.

The Reed-Frost approach, an attempt to resolve problems of random mixing and the meaning of transmission coefficients, uses the probability-of-contact concept:

$$C_{t+1} = S_t\{1 - (1 - p)C_t\}$$

where C_{t+1} and S_t are similar to the mass-action models and
p = the probability of contact necessary for infection.

Actually, in this model p is similar to the secondary-contact concept. These formulations have led to the development of chain binomial models that help us understand limited population groups where incubation and latent periods can be reconstructed, the classic effect being that of Greenwood.[21] With binomial trials, Greenwood expressed this relationship:

$$\text{Prob } (C_{t+1}|C_t, S_t) = \frac{S_t!}{C_{t+1}!S_{t+1}!} p^{(t+1)}(1 - p)^{S_t+1}$$

where p = probability of infection during serial interval.

Serial interval in this instance is the lag between primary and secondary cases. The Greenwood model has been successfully applied to limited population groups.

At the community level, the most successful models have been developed by Elveback and her co-workers over the past fifteen years.[22] Progressive adaptations of the Reed-Frost model have led to a better understanding of how influenza spreads within heterogeneous communities. Epidemics have been simulated for communities up to 1,000 persons that consider age, family size, and mixing pattern. Included are such aspects as the length of the latent period, the infective period and probabilities of contact, infection, and illness. These studies have been recently summarized by Elveback, and a simplified version of the basic model can be stated:[23]

$$Z_i = \sum_{g=1}^{G} S_i \, Pig \sum_{c=1}^{C} \theta_c$$

where Z_i = number of cases
$\quad S_i$ = susceptibility of person i
$\quad G$ = number of mixing groups
$\quad Pig$ = contact rate, person i in group g
$\quad C_g$ = number of infectives in group g
$\quad \theta_c$ = relative infectiousness of case c.

The overall procedure is highly detailed, and applications to large populations are not realistic because of the number of computations involved. As stated by Elveback, most models of a community epidemic still rely on some sort of transmissibility factor. In addition, the models normally used tend to begin with *one* infectious individual who actually starts the epidemic. Applications of influenza-simulation models to large populations—an entire country with many units of observation, for example—are still being refined.

Soviet researchers have been working on large-population influenza-diffusion models since the late 1960s. Based on daily morbidity reports from more than 100 large urban areas (more than 100,000 population), a continuous-time mass-action formulation has been put forth.[24] While numerous formulations have been published over the last fifteen years, the following sets of equations have been used repeatedly. Given city i:

$$\frac{dx_i}{dt} = \sum_{j=1}^{n} \left\{ \frac{\sigma_{ji}}{p_j} x_j - \frac{\sigma_{ij}}{p_i} x_i \right\} - \Phi(t, t);$$

$$\Phi(t, t) = \frac{\beta x_i \, y_i}{p_i} = \frac{\beta x_i}{p_i} \int_0^\infty \Phi_i(t, t - \tau)g(\tau) \, d\tau;$$

$$y_i(t) = \int_0^\infty \Phi_i(t, t - \tau)g(\tau) \, d\tau$$

where x = number of susceptibles
     y = number of cases
     λ = transmission factor
Φ (t,t) = number of new cases per time unit (one day)
  g (τ) = duration of cases
    P_i = population
    σij = a "migration term" (sometimes $P_i \, P_j^{2*-32}$)

As with the models already discussed, the Rvachev-Baroyan model uses a transmission factor (λ), and it assumes the typical shape of a given influenza cycle. Unlike some Western models, it includes urban population and assumes that it does not vary from one city to another. Population interaction is handled through the "migration" factor (σ_{ij}), but, curiously, distances among cities are not considered. Since larger cities are mostly used, the model can be utilized to predict the rate of increase for a given place during an epidemic, after initial seeding.

In an application of the model developed by the Soviet influenza researchers, Spicer was able to determine estimates of the time when an epidemic peak might be reached in England and Wales, as well as the overall size of an epidemic.[25] As explained by Spicer, the underlying philosophical basis of the model is the same as that proposed by McKendrick in 1927. One feature of the model that has drawn much attention is that the parameter (λ) used to simulate influenza diffusion is the same for every city. Simply stated:

$$R = \lambda \, SI$$

where R = incidence of new cases
     S = concentrations of susceptibles
     I = concentrations of immunes
and λ = the average number of new cases produced by a single infectious individual.

Since the Soviet model is based on continuous data and most countries with adequate reporting use forms of P&I mortality, Spicer has proposed a discrete form:

$$y_t + 1 = \lambda x_t \sum_{\tau=0}^{t} y_t - \tau \psi_\tau$$

$$X_{t+1} = x_t - y_{t+1}$$

where x_t = susceptible individuals at time t
y_t = new cases at time ti
ψ_τ = probability that a person is still infectious at time t after illness
and λ = transmissibility factor.

In practice, Spicer has worked out the following steps:

t	*number still infectious*
0	y_0
1	$y_1 \quad y_0 x_0$
2	$y_2 \quad y_1 x_0 \quad y_0 x_1$
3	$y_3 \quad y_2 x_0 \quad y_1 x_1 \quad y_0 x_2$

t	*susceptibles*
0	x_0
1	$x_0 - y_0 = x_1$
2	$x_0 - y_0 - y_1 = x_2$
3	$x_0 - y_0 - y_1 - y_2 = x_3$

t	*new cases*
1	$y_1 = \lambda x_0 y_0 \psi_0$
2	$y_2 = \lambda x_1 (y_1 \psi_0 + y_0 \psi_1)$
3	$y_3 = \lambda x_2 (y_2 \psi_0 + y_1 \psi_1 + y_0 \psi_2)$

Spicer fitted the model to data from England and Wales for epidemics taking place from 1958 to 1973 and found that it has a tendency to overpredict initially and wane before the actual data. This could be a reflection of a common pattern of underreporting at the onset of an influenza epidemic.

The two most important features that emerge from the conventional epidemiological approaches are populations of centers, or the "mass" of susceptibles and distance. The statistical testing in Chapter 7 indicated that distance-decay associations with surveillance city data for the United States can be identified particularly for the area east of the 100th meridian. Other distance-related associations are less clear. A method proposed by Zeller and Brown, operating on the assumption that a multinodal diffusion model utilizing population and distance might help explain influenza-spread patterns in the United States, is tested here.[26]

In the form of a Markov Chain–based computer program, SIMMAR has been adapted to report P&I mortality over six epidemics. The model considers two formulations:

$$A(t + 1) = A(t) + S(t)P^1(t)G(t + 1)F^{-1}$$

$$S_{it} = \frac{(a_{it}f_{ii})}{\Sigma(a_{it}f_{ii})}$$

where: $A(t)$ = a vector with elements a_{it} that are proportions of place i's population reporting influenza-pneumonia mortality by time t.

$S(t)$ = a vector with elements S_{it} that are proportions representing the number of cases in place i by time t relative to the total number of cases in all observed places at time t

P = a matrix with elements P_{ij} that represent the probability of transition from place i to place j

$p^1(t)$ = a matrix of transition probabilities adjusted to reflect nonvictims in place j at time t

$G(t+1)$ = a scalar representing the total number of new victims in time $t+1$

F = a diagonal matrix with elements f_{ii} that represent the population of each place i

Upon implementation of the model, the following modification is required:

$$A(t + 1) = A(t) + S^*(t)G(t + 1)F^{-2}$$

where $\quad S^*_{it} = \dfrac{\sum S_{it}P_{ij}(1 - a_{jt})}{\sum_i \sum_j S_{it}P_{jj}(1 - a_{jt})}$

This adjustment is made because the gross effect of deaths in all i places upon the population of i at time t is $\Sigma s_{it} P_{ij}$. Since a $_{it}$ is already infected, the net effect is reduced by $a - 1_{jt}$. The net effect in place j is S*jt.

In order to account for distance and the characteristic logistic shape of accumulated influenza during an epidemic, a gravity-model formulation ($P_{ij} = f_{ii} f_{ij}/d_{ij}^{\alpha}$), with d_{ij} as distance from i to j and α as a constant was used along with $G(t) = K/(1 + at^{-b})$, with K as the upper limit of the number of cases. This formulation adds the distance measure missing from the Soviet models.

The effects of summer fluctuations were removed by assuming that the "main wave" of any given epidemic did not begin until there was a clearly defined and steady increase in reporting during the late summer or autumn of each epidemic season. The available data for most years consist of the CDC weekly reports. The model was applied to such data, converted to rates, for the epidemics of 1928–29, 1943–44, 1947–48, 1968–69, 1977–78, and 1980–81. Overall variance was determined with the following results for the U.S. city sample groups:

Epidemic Season	R^2
1928–29	.715
1943–44	.780
1947–48	.759
1968–69	.826
1977–78	.675
1980–81	.684

The model, accounting for approximately 65 to 80 percent of the variance, indeed works best for multinodal epidemics, particularly the kind that transpired during the 1968–69 season. This is further proof that mass and distance are significant factors in influenza diffusion.

Comparisons of epidemics caused by presumably related H1N1 viruses indicated that this method tends to overpredict for larger cities and underpredict in south-central parts of the country. Also, there are differences between "expected" and actual rates from one epidemic to another and from one part of the country to another. Figures 8.10 to 8.13 represent a sampling of cities over four epidemics. As shown in Figure 8.10, the model underpredicted for Boston in three of four episodes, but, as shown in Figure 8.11, the model was more accurate for Washington, D.C., in three of four epidemics. There were substantial differences between observed and expected rates in St. Louis (Fig. 8.12), and the San Francisco results indicate consistently higher expectations than actual deaths. Other observa-

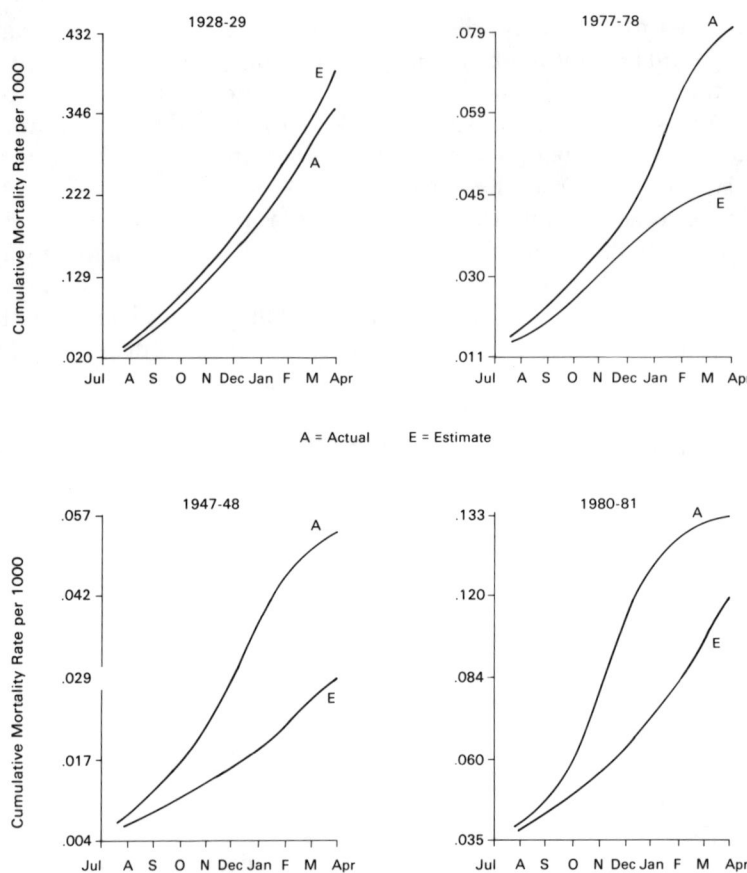

Figure 8.10. Comparisons of actual (A) and expected (E) influenza rates during four epidemics presumed to have been caused by related viral strains, using a simulation model based on a gravity-type formulation.

tions within this work support the latter results: West Coast influenza rates tend to be less than expected on the basis of national averages.

While the SIMMAR results are initially encouraging, the method is more appropriate for explaining the probable diffusion of endemic strains of influenza than the spread of newly introduced epidemic types of the disease. The addition of the gravity-model constraint underscores the importance of population mass and distance. Other

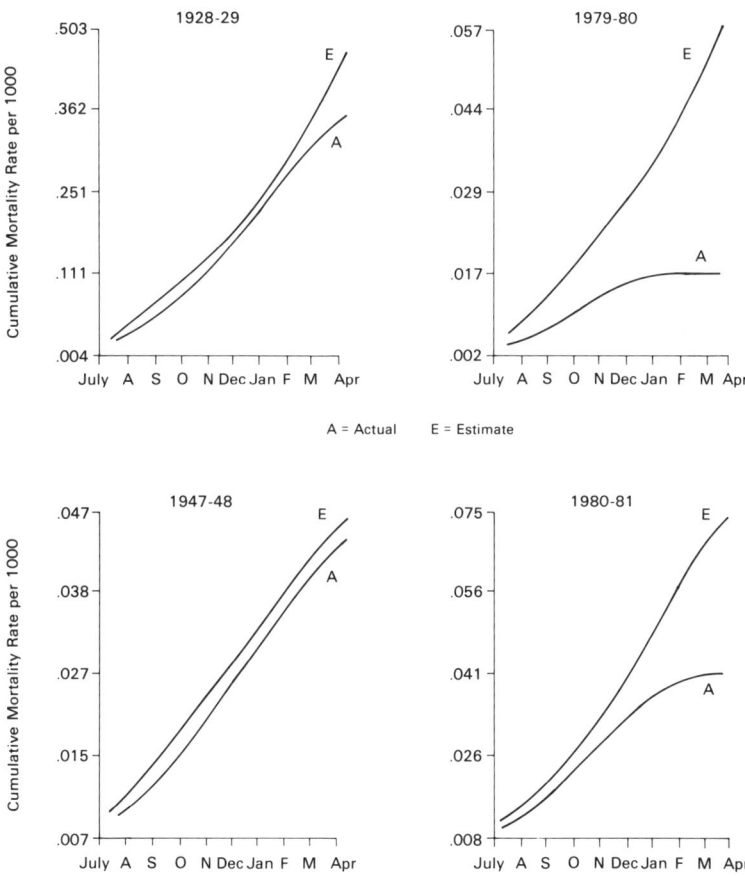

Figure 8.11. Actual (A) and expected (E) influenza deaths in Boston.

examinations of gravity-related models in regional science have also indicated that distance and attraction of mass can be even better understood by using a "potential" derivation of the family of models.[27] Given the importance of the elderly population as the highest-risk group during an epidemic, it can be shown in regression testing that an "elderly population potential" variable helps explain numbers of influenza deaths during different time priods. A typical application of this procedure would be to determine first the elderly population potential during the period t_1 taken in the example below [as 1980] in the following manner:

$$\sum_{i=1}^{181} \frac{E_j}{d_{ij}^2} * K$$

where E = population over 65
d_{ij} = distance between cities
K = potential of a city on itself.

The 181 unit areas utilized consist of the BEA (Bureau of Economic Analysis) spheres of influence shown in Figure 8.14.[28] As noted in

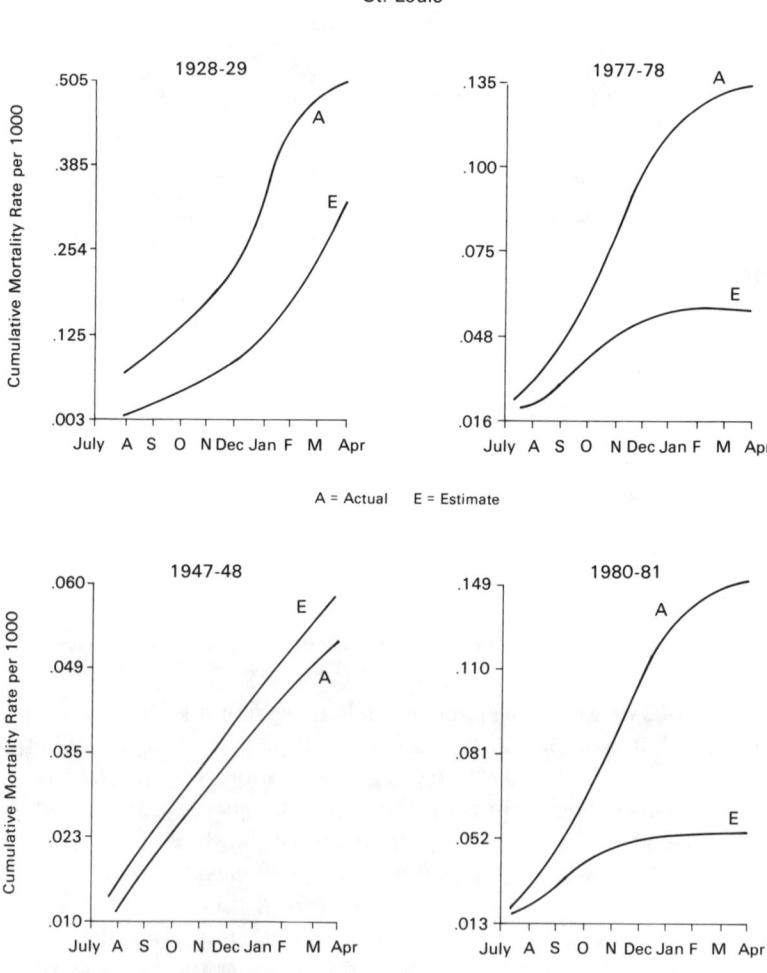

Figure 8.12. Actual (A) and expected (E) influenza deaths in St. Louis.

Chapter 7, any forecasting or simulation procedure would need to include all of the continental United States. The BEA spheres of influence are largely based on journey-to-work practices and thus representing one of the most accurate ways of determining urban nodal regions on the basis of what Berry terms the "Daily Urban System."[29] Elderly-population-potential measures were determined for each of the BEA unit areas, the these measures were used in a series of linear regressions as the independent variable. Dependent variables consisted of mortality counts for the 77 most statistically

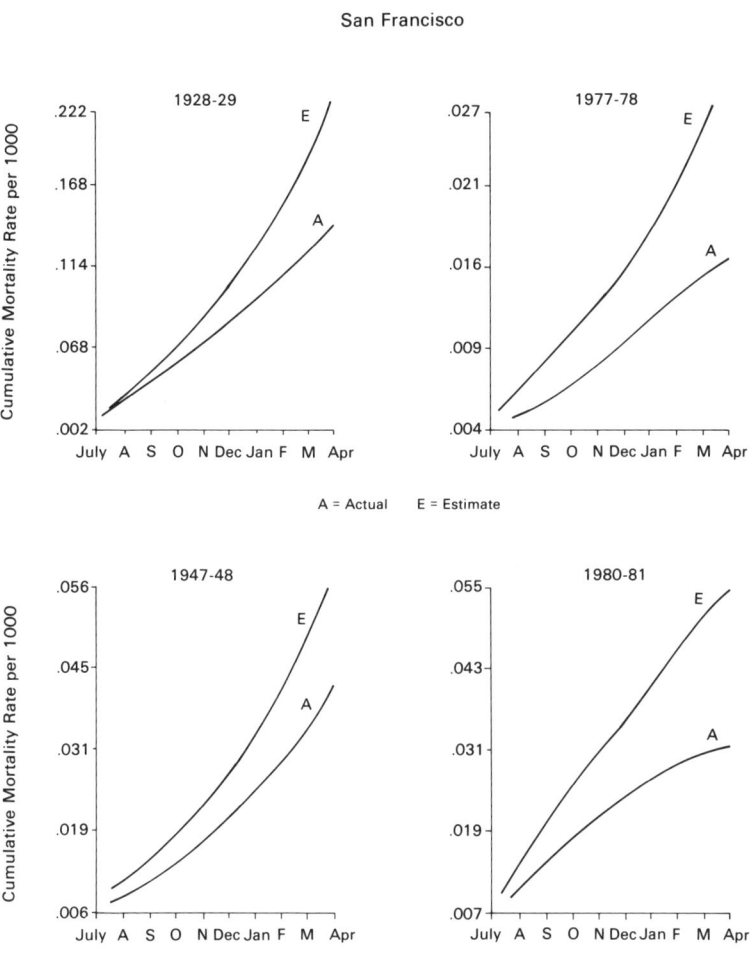

Figure 8.13. Comparisons of actual (A) and simulated (E) influenza mortality in San Francisco during four epidemics.

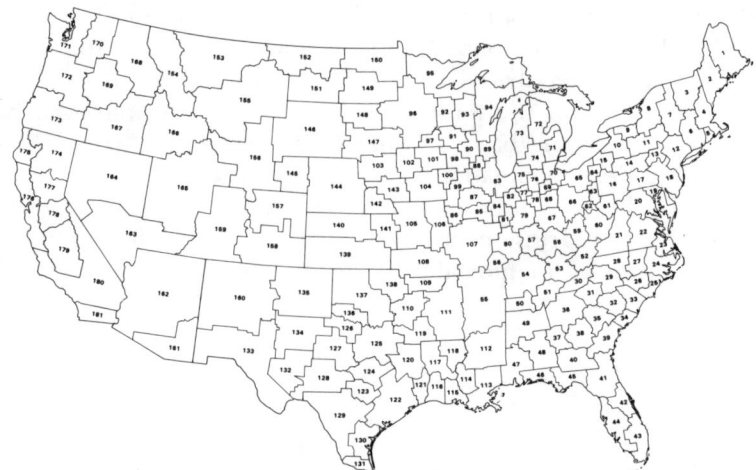

Figure 8.14. BEA unit areas recommended for future influenza diffusion studies.

significant cities shown in Figures 8.4 to 8.7, averaged from 1977 to 1984 by month. In spite of the differences in the determination of units of observation, at least half of the variance could be accounted for in most of the regressions.

It is also possible to "calibrate" the results of a specific regression and use the parameters (α) and (β) in an estimate of "expected" influenza cases during a specific month, assuming no changes in the prevailing strain of virus. The procedure is fairly straightforward.[30] First, 1990 elderly population potential can be determined using projections of the population over 65 years of age for the BEA unit areas.[31,32] The results of such a computation are shown in Figure 8.15. The 1980 regression parameters, α and β, were then applied to the forecasted 1990 population-potential measures to determine estimated influenza deaths by month. Figure 8.16 contains the results based on January reporting. The map could be entitled "any January, late 1980s," but it is based on the assumption that prevailing strains continue to cocirculate. The use of regressions demonstrates the importance of using the potential variant of the gravity model in estimating the possible future mortality of influenza, and at the same time the importance of the distribution of the elderly population is reemphasized. It can therefore be stated with a great deal of confidence that the most important ingredient in the simulation of influenza diffusion is the measure of the density of the elderly population and distance.

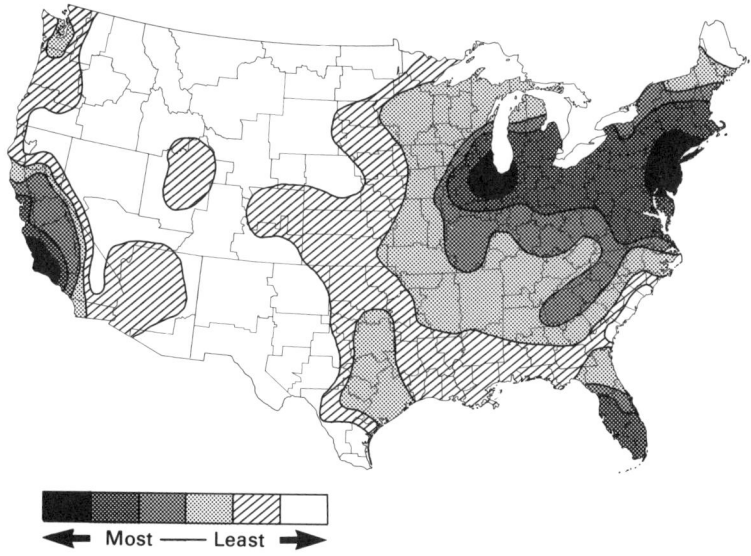

Figure 8.15. Elderly population potential projected to 1990, using BEA unit areas.

Simulated Alternative Diffusion Pathways

The literature on spatial diffusion is extensive. Works most pertinent to the simulation of influenza include the more recent contributions of Cliff et al.[33] and Brown,[34] although the latter work does not include considerations of disease; however, epidemiologists searching for definitive explanations to spatial-diffusion procedures should initially consult the long-standing expositions of Gould.[35] Gould's explanations of the attraction of population mass in relation to distance are equivalent to the epidemiological notions of "transmission factors." Such an interpretation is especially meaningful to developing an understanding of the simulation procedures suggested and applied by Hägerstrand and how they can be used in replicating influenza epidemics.[36] While the regression-based procedures in this chapter offer some clues to the probable distribution of future influenza deaths under the assumption that conditions remain constant and the SIMMAR gravity-model testing assists in understanding probably multicentered outbreaks, applications of Hägerstrand's basic modeling procedures offer the most viable alternatives in simulations of the spread of influenza if a new strain is introduced into a specific geographical area.

Hägerstrand's procedures in effect close the scale gap between

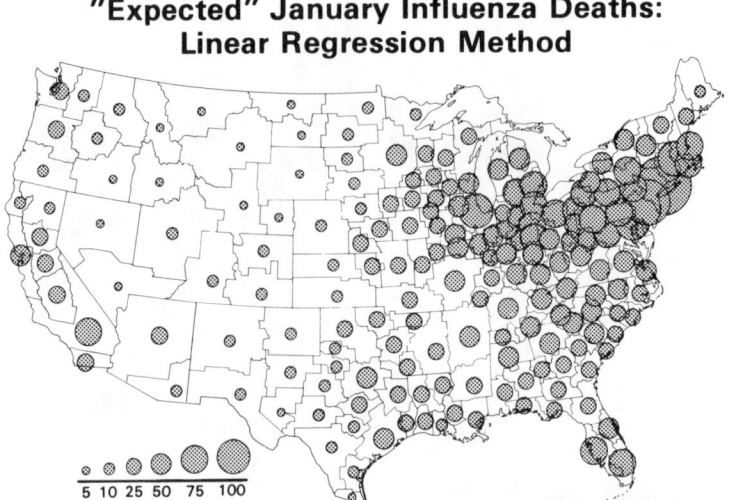

"Expected" January Influenza Deaths: Linear Regression Method

Figure 8.16. Even an uncomplicated linear regression model can give an approximation of expected influenza mortality during a specified period. This example might be labeled "Any January, late 1980s: All indicators constant."

conventional epidemiological-spread models and methods previously used in medical geography by the very nature of certain underlying assumptions. Most epidemiological models, with some exceptions, have not been effective for "communities" of more than 1,000 persons. Conversely, most disease-diffusion studies by geographers start with already-infected or about-to-be-infected communities and cities (see Chapter 1). Conceptually, the approaches advocated by Hägerstrand, and applied below, represent a smooth transition from the infected and contagious indivdual to an entire susceptible population.

The process begins with the notion that infected individuals are contained within cones of resolution based on distances from mathematical and geographical centers.[37] The probability of infection during an outbreak increases geometrically from the first contagious individual to others within groups of variable density. The rate of infection depends upon the virulence of a particular virus and specific levels of immunity, and operational procedures can replicate these conditions. More extensive cones of resolution, depending upon the size of areas and the amount of scale detail used, are expressed as mean information fields (MIFs), with the highest probabilities of infection in the centers. The MIF is operationalized in the form of a square grid with twenty-five cells (see Fig. 8.17). Probabilities of infection decrease with distance away from the centermost cell,

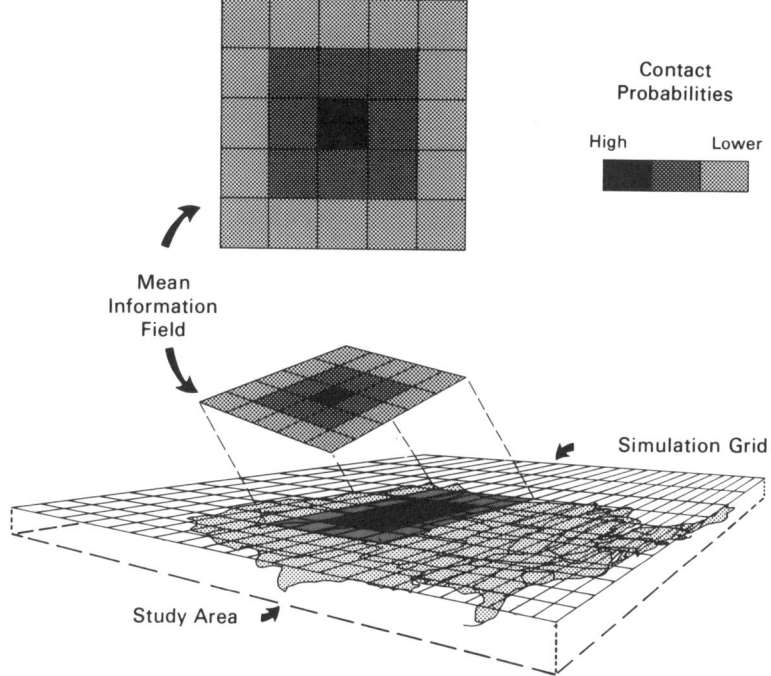

Figure 8.17. By converting the BEAs into a rectangular grid system, Hägerstrand's techniques can be applied to influenza-simulation models.

and in actual applications rates of differing distance-decay decrease can be expressed as different probabilities. The MIF is, in turn, "floated" over each of the cells within a more extensive geographical area covered by a simulation grid. On the basis of reported early cases of influenza, particularly new strains, the MIF stops floating. Random numbers, usually four-digit, are generated and matched with accumulated probabilities within the cells of the MIF. Since probabilities of contact are increasingly lower outward from the MIF center (cone of resolution), disease-diffusion probabilities correspond. The MIF continues to float and scan for new outbreak centers over successive interactions as infection also spreads outward from initial epicenters. In a specific procedure known as the Monte Carlo technique, epidemics can thus be simulated.

While various partial and more complete barriers of both human and natural origin can be added to the modeling process, the alternative simulations developed here are intended as examples of application and hence do not include barriers. Under other circumstances

Simulation Based on Random Origins

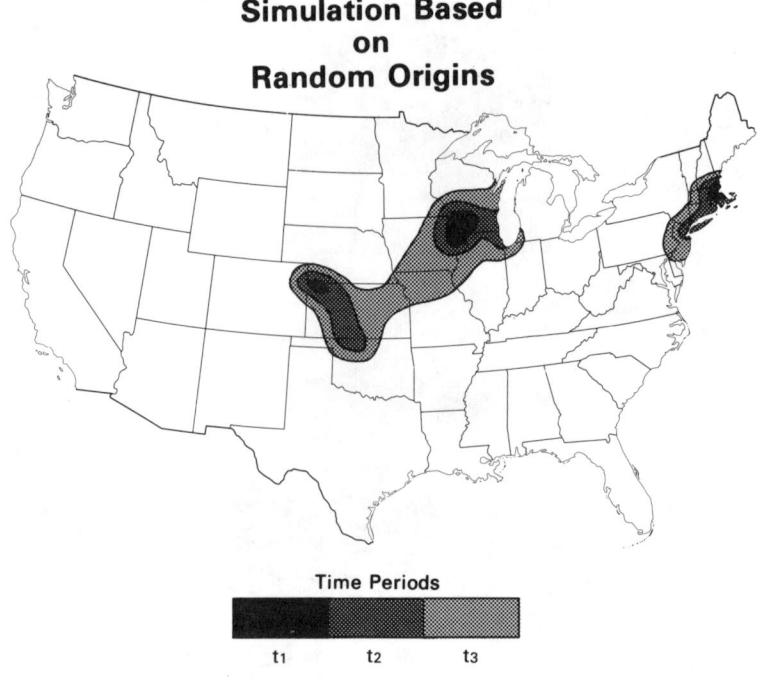

Time Periods

t1   t2   t3

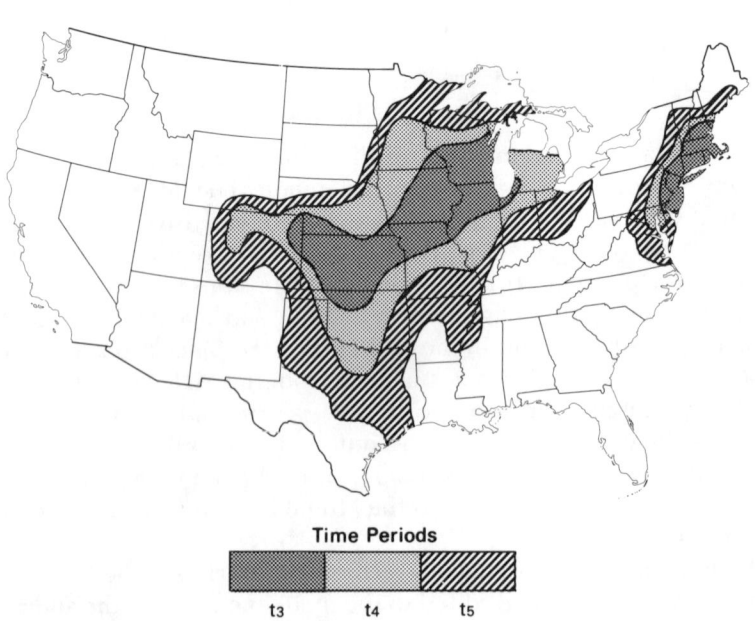

Time Periods

t3   t4   t5

Figure 8.18 These simulated influenza diffusion patterns were based on random points of origin.

Simulation Based
on
Random Origins

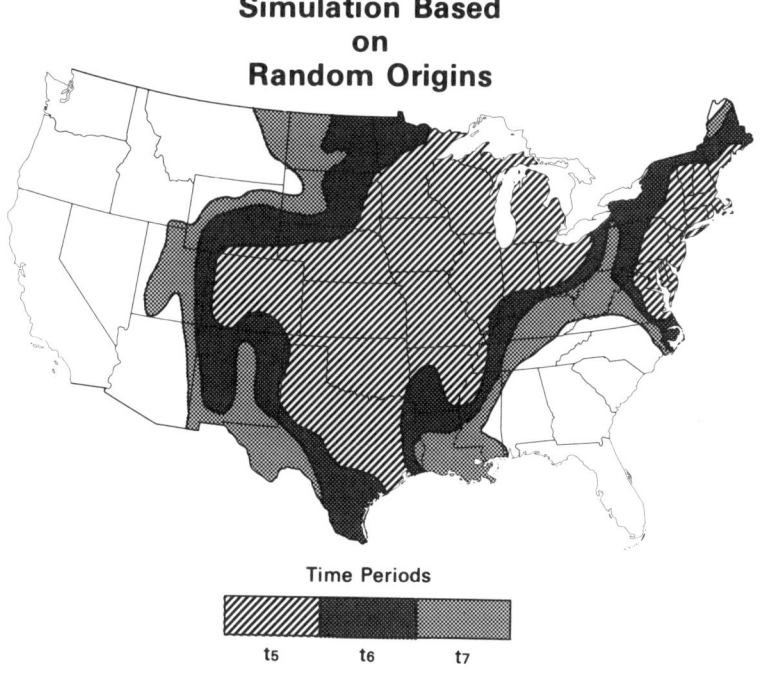

Time Periods

t5   t6   t7

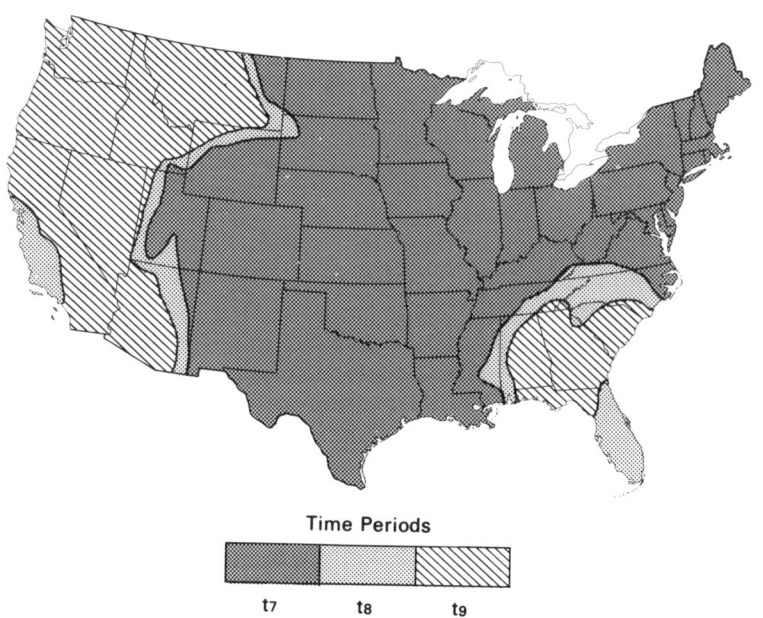

Time Periods

t7   t8   t9

Figure 8.19. Even random origins lead to infection of the
entire country.

the researcher may find it more appropriate to include such obstacles to influenza diffusion; however, the most comprehensive barriers consist of disease-prevention measures. For the examples depicted in Figures 8.18 to 8.23, the 181 BEA unit areas were converted to cells within a grid covering the entire United States. Within the cells the projected 1990 population over 65 years of age was used as the measure for mass of attraction. Since our knowledge of the spread of influenza over several decades indicates that rarely will only one place recognize the earliest infection, multiple centers have been selected for initial outbreaks. Numbers of influenza cases were then assigned on the basis of population. In three sets of twelve (monthly) iterations, origins have been determined by random selection—the urban hierarchy and "repeated events" (harmonic averages), respectively.

The results of a sequence of random-origins simulations are shown in Figures 8.18 and 8.19. The origins were selected on the basis of five random draws matched to cell numbers within the United States. Such a procedure can satisfy the assumption that an influenza epidemic can begin anywhere. Clearly, subsequent random draws would result in an epidemic with different epicenters. As shown in the maps, epicenters in the central parts of the country quickly coalesce as the epidemic also spreads up and down the Eastern Seaboard. Areas of infection eventually join up as the epidemic continues.

Following the theoretical assumption that an influenza epidemic would have a tendency to diffuse through the urban hierarchy even with random origins, the successive iterations expressed in Figures 8.20 and 8.21 were developed. Borchert's first- and second-order centers were used as the basis for early infections within major centers of the urban hierarchy.[38] Note, then, that the traditional Manufacturing Belt and the Gulf and West coasts are quickly infected, and by the fifth iteration ($t = 5$), Denver would emerge as an island of infection. This hierarchical alternative further suggests that influenza would continue to spread through the urban system in a manner somewhat similar to the results obtained from regressions using population potential as an independent variable. Since most epidemics of influenza have not been truly hierarchical in diffusion over many episodes that probably did not include the introduction of a new strain of the disease, the third alternative was selected.

Referred to here as the "repeated events" alternative, the seven earliest areas of outbreak based on the patterns of the winter seasons extending from 1977–78 to 1983–84 were used as locations of epidemic origin. The cells were identified on the basis of the results of harmonic analysis: Peak months were converted from radians determined from seasonal averages for the entire time period. These origins are shown in Figure 8.22. For some reasons not fully understood, these places have reported influenza outbreaks in recent years earlier than others. The diffusion pattern that emerges is partially hierarchical, and, by the very nature of the method, partially random. Still, in a few time periods, central portions of the country are rapidly infected along with the Northeast and Florida. Eventually, the simulated epidemic spreads to the Pacific Northwest and then California.

These alternative simulations are intended as examples of how Hägerstrand's approach can be used in the simulation of influenza. Clearly, repeated simulations would be required under actual epidemic circumstances, but the utility of the approach cannot be underestimated as the first choice in modeling the diffusion of influenza. The three alternatives developed above all emerge as "characteristic" epidemic curves when cumulative proportions of mortality are compared with time spans (see Fig. 8.24). As would be expected, the random-origins alternative resulted in a slightly slower rate of infection in this instance. In actuality, true rates of spread depend upon the type of virus that is introduced.

Spatial Aspects of Prevention and Control

In May 1985 the Immunization Practices Advisory Committee (ACIP) of the U.S. Public Health Service issued an updated statement pertaining to routes of vaccine administration and alternative methods of prophylaxis.[39] Specifically, immediate attention was given to the use of amantadine hydrochloride as a short-term option to inactivated vaccine. Such a barrier to the diffusion of influenza would be particularly important if a new strain of influenza were to emerge and vaccine were in short supply, if immediately available at all. Clearly, immunization is still the most viable alternative to control, and specific target groups continue to be persons with severe chronic disorders, residents of nursing homes and other institutions, medical personnel, healthy people over 65, and others who think they need an inoculation. Recognition of the "elderly population potential" variable is obvious for both control alternatives.

As would also unfortunately be expected, no mention was made of any geographical strategies that might be included, particularly if an emergency situation were to arise. One of the major purposes of this book is to offer such an additional spatial ingredient in prevention and control efforts. Once initial outbreaks of a new strain are identified, spatial-simulation procedures as outlined in this chapter should be added to any medical control efforts. Of course, it would take repeated iterations of the simulation procedure at several different scales than are used in the example presented here. In addition,

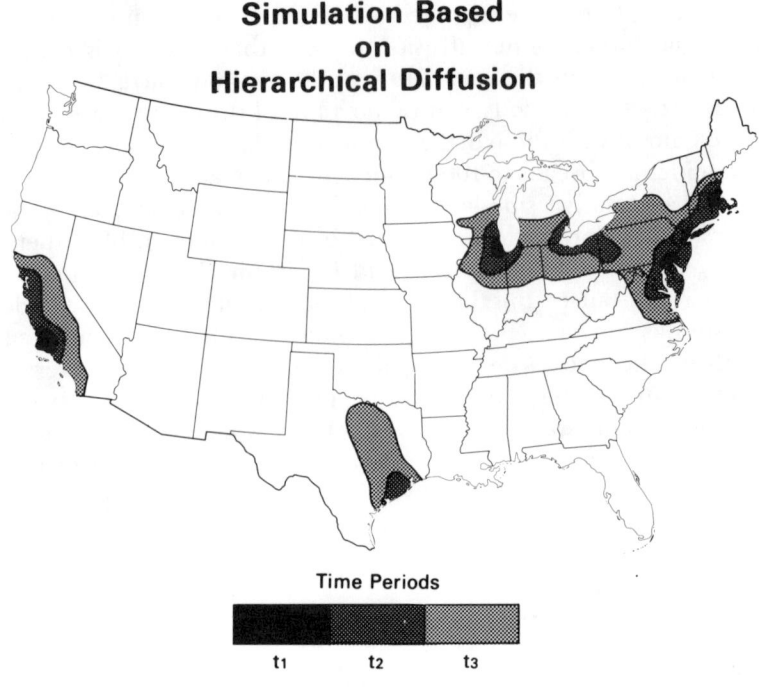

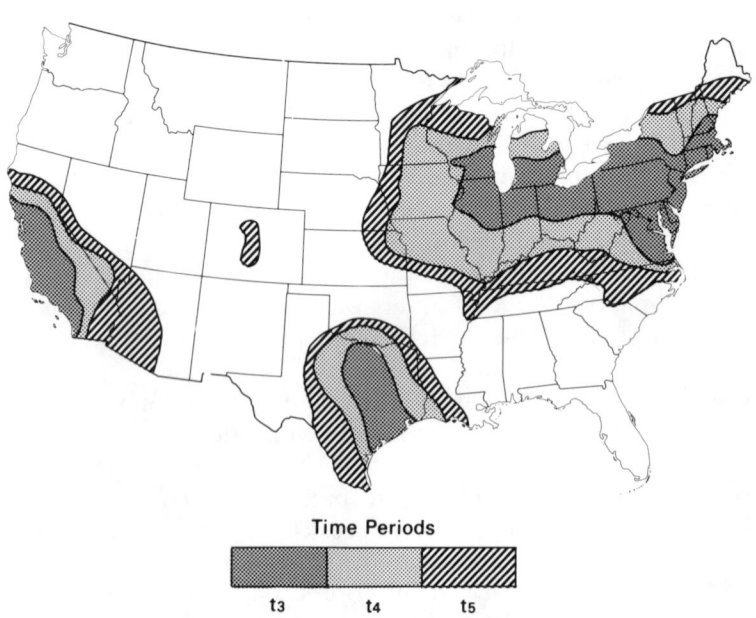

Figure 8.20. We could expect diffusion patterns similar to these if rank-size relationships have anything to do with the spread of influenza.

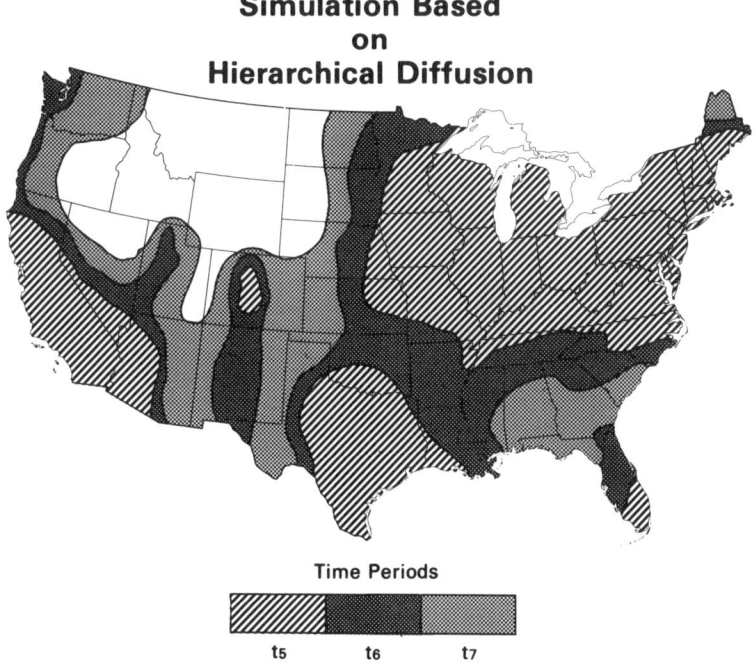

Figure 8.21. Saturation due to hierarchical diffusion.

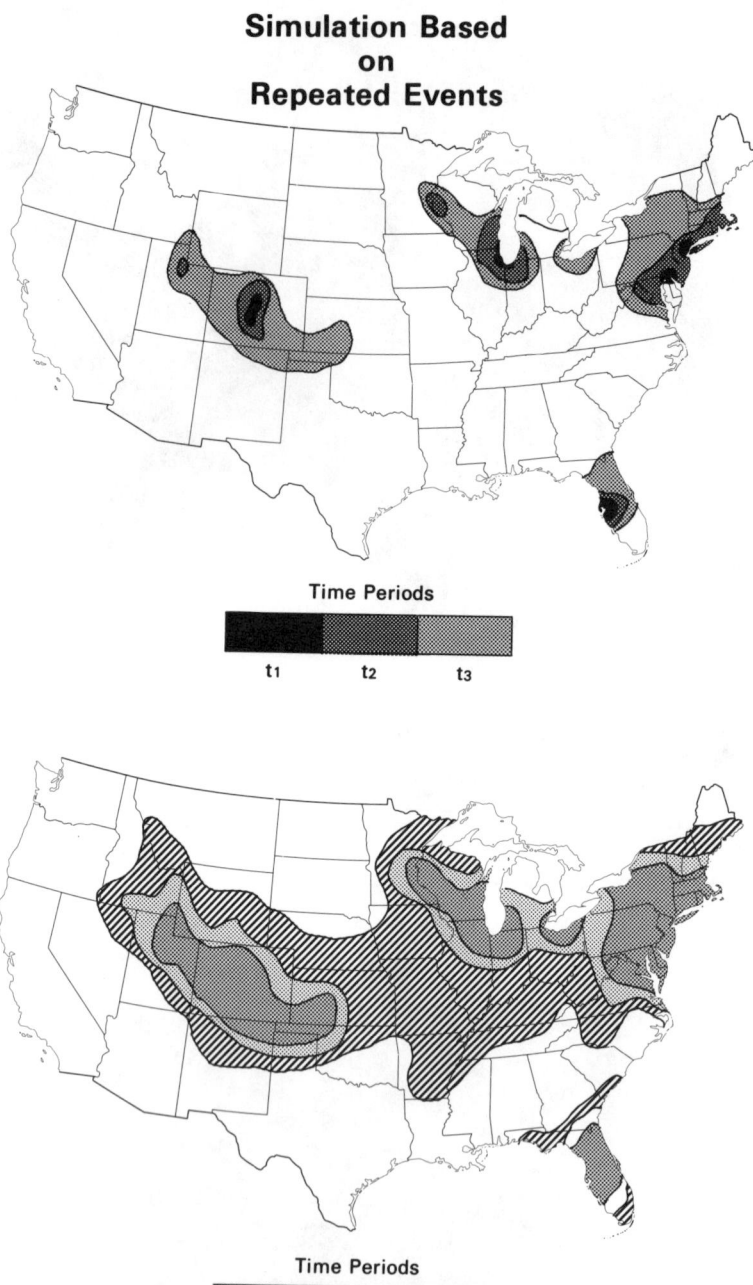

Figure 8.22. These simulated influenza diffusion patterns result from using harmonic averages to determine points of origin.

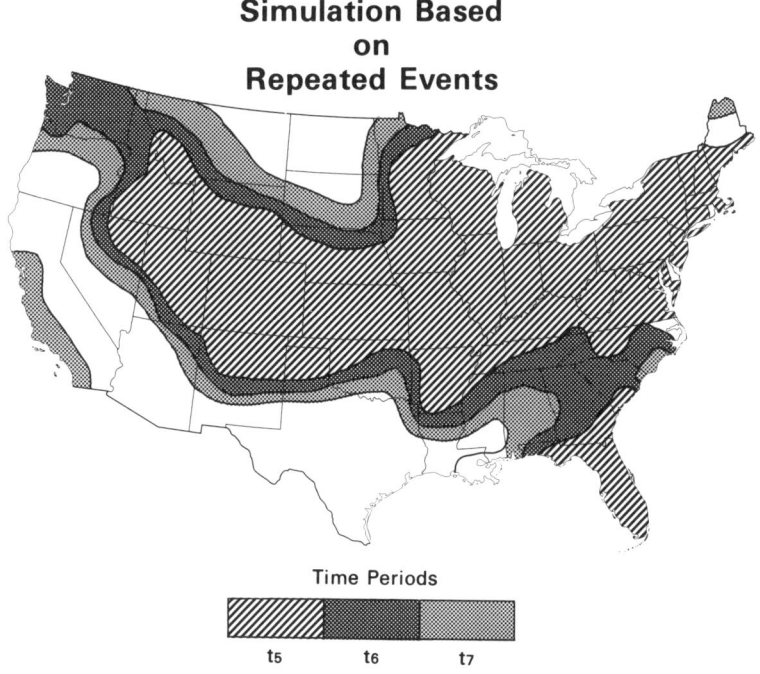

Figure 8.23. Saturation-phase diffusion using harmonic origins.

Table 8.3   BEA Economic Areas, 1985

1. Bangor, Maine
2. Portland–Lewiston, Maine
3. Burlington, Vt.
4. Boston, Mass.
5. Providence–Warwick–Pawtucket, R.I.
6. Hartford–New Haven–Springfield, Conn.–Mass.
7. Albany–Schenectady–Troy, N.Y.
8. Syracuse–Utica, N.Y.
9. Rochester, N.Y.
10. Buffalo, N.Y.
11. Binghamton–Elmira, N.Y.
12. New York, N.Y.
13. Scranton–Wilkes-Barre, Pa.
14. Williamsport, Pa.
15. Erie, Pa.
16. Pittsburgh, Pa.
17. Harrisburg–York–Lancaster, Pa.
18. Philadelphia, Pa.
19. Baltimore, Md.
20. Washington, D.C.
21. Roanoke–Lynchburg, Va.
22. Richmond, Va.
23. Norfolk–Virginia Beach–Newport News, Va.
24. Rocky Mount–Wilson–Greenville, N.C.
25. Wilmington, N.C.
26. Fayetteville, N.C.
27. Raleigh–Durham, N.C.
28. Greensboro–Winston-Salem–High Point, N.C.
29. Charlotte, N.C.
30. Asheville, N.C.
31. Greenville–Spartanburg, S.C.
32. Columbia, S.C.
33. Florence, S.C.
34. Charleston–North Charleston, S.C.
35. Augusta, Ga.
36. Atlanta, Ga.
37. Columbus, Ga.
38. Macon, Ga.
39. Savannah, Ga.
40. Albany, Ga.
41. Jacksonville, Fla.
42. Orlando–Melbourne–Daytona Beach, Fla.
43. Miami–Fort Lauderdale, Fla.

44. Tampa–St. Petersburg, Fla.
45. Tallahassee, Fla.
46. Pensacola–Panama City, Fla.
47. Mobile, Ala.
48. Montogmery, Ala.
49. Birmingham, Ala.
50. Huntsville–Florence, Ala.
51. Chattanooga, Tenn.
52. Johnson City–Kingsport–Bristol, Tenn.–Va.
53. Knoxville, Tenn.
54. Nashville, Tenn.
55. Memphis, Tenn.
56. Paducah, Tenn.
57. Louisville, Ky.
58. Lexington, Ky.
59. Huntington, W.Va.
60. Charleston, W.Va.
61. Morgantown–Fairmont, W.Va.
62. Parkersburg, W.Va.
63. Wheeling–Steubenville–Weirton, W.Va.–Ohio
64. Youngstown-Warren, Ohio
65. Cleveland, Ohio
66. Columbus, Ohio
67. Cincinnati, Ohio
68. Dayton, Ohio
69. Lima, Ohio
70. Toledo, Ohio
71. Detroit, Mich.
72. Saginaw Bay–Bay City, Mich.
73. Grand Rapids, Mich.
74. Lansing–Kalamazoo, Mich.
75. South Bend, Ind.
76. Fort Wayne, Ind.
77. Kokomo–Marion, Ind.
78. Anderson–Muncie, Ind.
79. Indianapolis, Ind.
80. Evansville, Ind.
81. Terra Haute, Ind.
82. Lafayette, Ind.
83. Chicago, Ill.
84. Champaign-Urbana, Ill.
85. Springfield–Decatur, Ill.
86. Quincy, Ill.
87. Peoria, Ill.
88. Rockford, Ill.
89. Milwaukee, Wis.
90. Madison, Wis.

91. La Cross, Wis.
92. Eau Claire, Wis.
93. Wausau, Wis.
94. Appleton–Green Bay–Oshkosh, Wis.
95. Duluth, Minn.
96. Minneapolis–St. Paul, Minn.
97. Rochester, Minn.
98. Dubuque, Iowa
99. Davenport–Rock Island–Moline, Iowa–Ill.
100. Cedar Rapids, Iowa
101. Waterloo, Iowa
102. Fort Dodge, Iowa
103. Sioux City, Iowa
104. Des Moines, Iowa
105. Kansas City, Mo.
106. Columbia, Ohio
107. St. Louis, Mo.
108. Springfield, Mo.
109. Fayetteville, Ark.
110. Fort Smith, Ark.
111. Little Rock–North Little Rock, Ark.
112. Jackson, Miss.
113. New Orleans, La.
114. Baton Rouge, La.
115. Lafayette, La.
116. Lake Charles, La.
117. Shreveport, La.
118. Monroe, La.
119. Texarkana, Tex.
120. Tyler-Longview, Tex.
121. Beaumont-Port Arthur, Tex.
122. Houston, Tex.
123. Austin, Tex.
124. Waco–Killeen–Temple, Tex.
125. Dallas-Fort Worth, Tex.
126. Wichita Falls, Tex.
127. Abilene, Tex.
128. San Angelo, Tex.
129. San Antonio, Tex.
130. Corpus Christi, Tex.
131. Brownsville–McAllen–Harlingen, Tex.
132. Odessa–Midland, Tex.
133. El Paso, Tex.
134. Lubbock, Tex.
135. Amarillo, Tex.
136. Lawton, Okla.
137. Oklahoma City, Okla.
138. Tulsa, Okla.
139. Wichita, Kans.
140. Salina, Kans.
141. Topeka, Kans.
142. Lincoln, Nebr.
143. Omaha, Nebr.
144. Grand Island, Nebr.
145. Scottsbluff, Nebr.
146. Rapid City, S.Dak.
147. Sioux Falls, S.Dak.
148. Aberdeen, S.Dak.
149. Fargo–Moorhead, N.Dak.–Minn.
150. Grand Forks, N.Dak.
151. Bismarck, N.Dak.
152. Minot, N.Dak.
153. Great Falls, Mont.
154. Missoula, Mont.
155. Billings, Mont.
156. Cheyenne–Casper, Wyo.
157. Denver, Colo.
158. Colorado Springs–Pueblo, Colo.
159. Grand Junction, Colo.
160. Albuquerque, N.Mex.
161. Tucson, Ariz.
162. Phoenix, Ariz.
163. Las Vegas, Nev.
164. Reno, Nev.
165. Salt Lake City–Ogden, Utah
166. Pocatello–Idaho Falls, Idaho
167. Boise City, Idaho
168. Spokane, Wash.
169. Richland, Wash.
170. Yakima, Wash.
171. Seattle, Wash.
172. Portland, Oreg.
173. Eugene, Oreg.
174. Redding, Calif.
175. Eureka, Calif.
176. San Francisco–Oakland–San Jose, Calif.
177. Sacramento, Calif.
178. Stockton–Modesto, Calif.
179. Fresno–Bakersfield, Calif.
180. Los Angeles, Calif.
181. San Diego, Calif.
182. Anchorage, Alaska
183. Honolulu, Hawaii

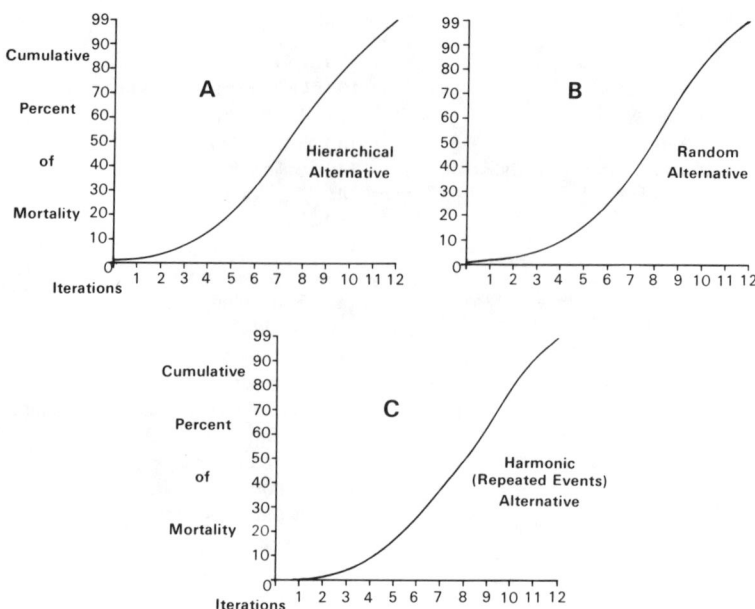

Figure 8.24. These comparisons of the cumulative effects of simulated diffusion show numerical trends more similar than the geographical patterns, and this circumstance has plagued many influenza researchers over the past seventy years.

probabilities would have to be periodically and speedily recalibrated. However, all of this can be accomplished in short order given current computer technologies. It would be simple to identify diffusion pathways and target specific areas for immediate distribution of either a vaccine or amantadine. If geographical barriers can slow down the spread of influenza during a pandemic, an epidemic, or even a major outbreak, an important contribution will have been made. It is up to both the third generation of influenza public health workers and key elected officials to accept and use this spatial form of augmentation of disease prevention and control.

Notes

1. Centers for Disease Control, "Influenza Surveillance," Report No. 94. (Atlanta: U.S. Department of Health and Human Services, Public Health Service, June 1984).
2. Ibid., "Influenza Mortality Surveillance," *MMWR* 29 (December 5, 1980), pp. 578–80.

3. Ibid., "Influenza–U.S.S.R., Hong Kong," *MMWR* 26 (December 16, 1977), p. 410.
4. Ibid., "Influenza–Worldwide," *MMWR* 27 (February 3, 1978), p. 40.
5. Ibid., "Influenza–United States," *MMWR* 29 (January 2, 1981), pp. 615–16.
6. Ibid., "Antigenic Analysis of Influenza A Viruses," *MMWR* 30 (March 13, 1981), pp. 110–12.
7. Paul Schureman, *Manual of Harmonic Analysis and Prediction of Tides* (Washington, D.C.: U.S. Department of Commerce, Coast and Geodetic Survey, 1958).
8. L. H. Horn and R. A. Bryson, "Harmonic Analysis of the Annual March of Precipitation over the United States," *Annals, Association of American Geographers* 50 (1960), pp. 157–71.
9. Michael E. Sabbagh and Reid A. Bryson, "Aspects of the Precipitation Climatology of Canada Investigated by the Method of Harmonic Analysis," *Annals, Association of American Geographers* 52 (1962), pp. 426–60. Also reprinted as Chapter 10 in Brian J. L. Berry and Duane F. Marble, eds. *Spatial Analysis* (Englewood Cliffs, N.J.: 1968), pp. 250–65.
10. Charles M. Brooks and N. Carruthers, *Handbook of Statistical Methods in Meteorology* (London: Her Majesty's Stationery Office, 1953, 1967).
11. Glenn W. Brier, "Long-Range Prediction of the Zonal Westerlies and Some Problems in Data Analysis," *Reviews of Geophysics* 61 (1968), pp. 525–51.
12. Ibid., "The Quasi-Biennial Oscillation and Feedback Processes in the Atmosphere–Ocean–Earth System," *Monthly Weather Review* 106 (1978), pp. 938–46.
13. A. D. Cliff, P. Haggett, J. K. Ord, and G. R. Versey, *Spatial Diffusion: An Historical Geography of Epidemics in an Island Community* (Cambridge: Cambridge University Press, 1981).
14. L. R. Elveback et al., "An Influenza Simulation Model for Immunization Studies," *American Journal of Epidemiology* 103 (1976), pp. 152–65.
15. N. T. J. Bailey, *The Mathematical Theory of Infectious Diseases and Its Applications* (London: Charles Griffith, 1975). In addition, the 250,000 figure was discussed through personal communication in 1981.
16. O. V. Baroyan et al., "Computer Modeling of Influenza Epidemics for the Whole Country (U.S.S.R.)," *Advances in Applied Probability* 3 (1971), pp. 224–26.
17. Paul Fine, "Applications of Mathematical Models to the Epidemiology of Influenza: A Critique," in Philip Selby, ed., *Influenza Models: Prospects for Development and Use* (Lancaster, Boston, and The Hague: MTP Press, 1982), pp. 15–85.
18. J. M. Hunter and J. C. Young, "Diffusion of Influenza in England and Wales," *Annals, Association of American Geographers* 61 (December 1971), pp. 637–53.
19. L. A. Brown, *Innovation Diffusion: A New Perspective* (New York and London: Methuen, 1981); and Robert Q. Hanham and Lawrence A. Brown, "Diffusion Waves Within the Context of Regional Economic Development," *Journal of Regional Science* 16 (1976), pp. 65–71.
20. Paul E. M. Fine, "A Commentary on the Mechanical Analogue of the Reed-Frost Model," *American Journal of Epidemiology* 106 (1977), pp. 87–100.
21. M. Greenwood, "The Infectiousness of Measles," *Biometrika* 36 (1949), pp. 1–8.
22. L. R. Elveback, "Models of Family and Small Community Spread," in Philip Selby, ed., *Influenza Models*.
23. Ibid., p. 162.
24. Fine, "Applications of Mathematical Models."
25. Clive C. Spicer, "The Mathematical Modelling of Influenza Epidemics," *British Medical Bulletin* 35 (1979), pp. 23–28.
26. Richard E. Zeller and Lawrence A. Brown, "SIMMAR: A Markov Chain Based Program for the Diffusion of Innovation," Studies in the Diffusion of Innovation. Discussion Paper No. 7, Department of Geography, Ohio State University, 1970.
27. Lawrence A. Brown, John Odland, and Reginald G. Golledge, "Migration, Functional Distance, and the Urban Hierarchy," *Economic Geography* 46 (1970), pp. 472–85.
28. U.S. Department of Commerce, Social and Economic Statistics Administration, Bureau of Economic Analysis, "Area Economic Projections, 1990," Washington: U.S. Government Printing Office, Stock Number 003–024–00490–9, 1979.

29. Brian J. L. Berry, "Hierarchical Diffusion: The Basis of Developmental Filtering and Spread in a System of Growth Centers," in N. M. Hansen, ed., *Growth Centers in Regional Economic Development* (New York: The Free Press, 1972).
30. Gerald F. Pyle, *Heart Disease, Cancer and Stroke in Chicago* (Chicago: University of Chicago, Department of Geography, Research Monograph No. 134, 1971).
31. U.S. Department of Commerce, "Area Economic Projections, 1990."
32. U.S. Department of Commerce, Bureau of the Census, "Provisional Projections of the Population of States, by Age and Sex: 1980 to 2000," Population Estimates and Projections, Series P-25, No. 937, 1983.
33. Cliff et al., *Spatial Diffusion.*
34. Lawrence A. Brown, *Diffusion Processes and Location: A Conceptual Framework and Bibliography* (Philadelphia: Regional Science Research Institute, 1968).
35. Peter R. Gould, *Spatial Diffusion* (Washington, D.C.: Association of American Geographers, Resource Paper Series, No. 4, 1969).
36. Torsten Hägerstrand, *The Propagation of Innovation Waves*, Lund Studies in Geography, Series B, No. 4 (Lund: Gleerup, 1952).
37. Ronald Abler, John Adams, and Peter Gould, *Spatial Organization: The Geographer's View of the World* (Englewood Cliffs, N.J.: Prentice-Hall, 1971), pp. 389–451.
38. John R. Borchert, "America's Changing Metropolitan Regions," *Annals, Association of American Geographers* 62 (1972), pp. 352–71.
39. Centers for Disease Control, "Prevention and Control of Influenza," *MMWR* 3 (May 17, 1985), pp. 261–75.

Index

Date Due